The
Pregnant Woman's
Comfort Guide

Safe, Quick and Easy Relief
from the Discomforts of Pregnancy & Postpartum

The
Pregnant Woman's
Comfort Guide

Safe, Quick and Easy Relief
from the Discomforts of Pregnancy & Postpartum

Sherry LM Jiménez, RN

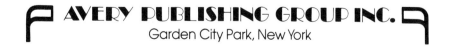
AVERY PUBLISHING GROUP INC.
Garden City Park, New York

The health procedures and exercises in this book are based upon the training, personal experience, and research of the author. Because each person and situation is unique, the author and publisher urge the reader to check with a qualified health professional before using any procedure where there is any question as to its appropriateness.

Cover designers: Small Kaps
In-house editor: Bonnie Freid
Typesetters: Widget Design
Inside artwork: Jan Antos and Widget Design

Library of Congress Cataloging-in-Publication Data

Jiménez, Sherry Lynn Mims.
    The pregnant woman's comfort guide: safe, quick, and easy relief
  from the discomforts of pregnancy & postpartum / Sherry L.M.
  Jiménez.
      p. cm.
    Includes index.
    ISBN 0-89529-490-7
    1. Pregnancy. 2. Pregnancy, Complications of. 3. Naturopathy.
  I. Title.
  RG525.J556   1992
  618.2′4—dc20   91-33379
                                                            CIP

Printed in the United States of America

10 9 8 7 6 5 4 3 2 1

Contents

Dedication

This book is dedicated to the mothers and fathers who read it, and to all babies – unborn and newborn – who, like their parents, are created in the image of God.

Acknowledgments

The Pregnant Woman's Comfort Guide, like most of the books and articles I've written, is based on the hard work and experience of thousands of expectant and new parents and, once again, I gratefully acknowledge their help. A very special thank you must go to the expectant mothers from my 1982 morning prenatal exercise class who first asked me for a book to deal with "all those nit-picky things of pregnancy."

I've also learned from and relied on the hard work and experiences of hundreds of maternal health professionals — nurse researchers, medical researchers, childbirth educators, midwives, and maternity nurses and physicians. I have worked with them, attended their lectures, read their books and articles, and shared with them the joy of serendipitous learning at conferences and workshops for organizations such as NAACOG, ACOG, ASPO/Lamaze, and ICEA.

I owe both my thanks and my appreciation to Sharron S. Humenick, R.N., Ph.D., F.A.A.N., Professor of Nursing at the University of Wyoming in Laramie. Sharron took me under her wing back in 1974. She encouraged me through the ASPO/Lamaze certification process for childbirth educators, held my hand through my first overnight trip away from my children, became my mentor as I found my own wings as a childbirth educator, and is my friend. I also want to acknowledge William Graves, M.D., F.A.C.O.G., and Robert Marcus, M.D., F.A.C.O.G. — two of the many obstetricians with whom I've worked who have helped make safe and satisfying family-centered maternity care a reality.

Thanks, too, go to my daughter, Amy Rebecca, who spent her summer typing the manuscript of the first edition of this book onto a computer disk, and to my son, Daniel, who rescued me from many traumatic tricks played by my computer. And I thank my husband, Angel R. Jimenez, M.D., F.A.C.S. — back in 1979 he believed I could write something and actually get it published. Since then, he's had doubts about the financial wisdom of my writing about pregnancy, but he has never stopped believing.

Finally, a belated thank you to Neil Diamond—his records and tapes provided the background music for my exercise and relaxation classes for many years and for every word I've written since 1980. All in all, it's been a "Beautiful Noise."

A Word About Gender

Your baby is certainly as likely to be a boy as a girl; however, our language does not provide us with a genderless pronoun. To avoid using the awkward "he/she" or the impersonal "it" when referring to your baby, while still giving equal time to both sexes, I have alternated the gender of personal pronouns throughout the book. Consequently, you will read "she" in some sections and "he" in others. This decision has been made in the interest of simplicity and clarity.

Preface

"Give us a book that shows us how to deal with all the nit-picky problems of pregnancy."

More than eight years ago, that unanimous challenge was presented to me by the members of my morning prenatal exercise class. The result of their challenge was the first edition of *The Pregnant Woman's Comfort Guide*, published in 1983. Now, eight years later, I'm answering a challenge from nurses and childbirth educators who have asked that the Comfort Guide be made available again for the expectant and new mothers with whom they work.

The Comfort Guide is based on a wholistic, comprehensive approach to childbearing. Although "wholistic" may sound like something out of New Age philosophy, it's not. In fact, it's an ancient philosophy that states that we were created with a body, a mind, and a spirit, all of which must live in harmony within us. When there is conflict within or among these, it causes distress, which often leads to pain or illness. A wholistic approach to childbearing takes each part into consideration when dealing with your distress. So, in the Comfort Guide, I'll ask you to consider many aspects of your life—your family, your marriage, your work, your hopes and fears, your way of eating or sleeping, and even your way of walking.

This second edition of the Comfort Guide covers all of the seventy-plus discomforts and changes of pregnancy and postpartum that were covered in the first edition; and there are still plenty of illustrations throughout the book. I've increased the focus on preventing discomforts and I've added a number of new comfort techniques, as well as several new topics, including postpartum grief and baby blues. You'll also notice some new features, such as tips for handling discomfort during labor, quotes from new and expectant parents, myths about pregnancy, and a few personal observations.

The comfort measures in this book are easy and practical and they all are based on three characteristics common to all the changes and discomforts of pregnancy and postpartum:

❏ They are legitimate.

❏ They are temporary.

❏ They can be relieved, or at least reduced, through natural, nonmedical means.

As you use these natural remedies to help yourself, you'll learn to take your problems and distress into your own hands and to deal effectively with them. You'll learn a new reaction to stress — instead of looking to someone or something else for relief, you'll learn to look to yourself. By the time you go into labor, your natural reaction to stress will be one of determination and action, not of passive acceptance and fear.

Whether you use this book as part of a prepared childbirth class or as your own guide through pregnancy and postpartum, you'll soon find that it does more than help you relieve your discomforts — it shows you how to keep yourself and your baby healthy and safe, and it helps you gain the energy and vitality you need during this special time called "childbearing."

How to Use This Book

The Comfort Guide is arranged in two parts. On pages 1 through 116, you'll learn how to cope with the changes and discomforts of pregnancy, and on pages 117 through 168, you'll learn how to handle the changes and discomforts of postpartum. Under each specific problem, you'll find a simple explanation of what causes it, followed by several easy and practical solutions. Be sure you don't skip over the explanation of what causes the problem. You'll need this information in order to make the best use of the advice that will follow.

In order to make the Comfort Guide easier to use, preventive tips and comfort measures for each situation are listed separately according to "What to Do" and "What to Avoid." Explanations and illustrations of exercises, massages, and relaxation techniques follow these lists.

In your Comfort Guide you'll discover a variety of ways to deal with the changes and discomforts of the childbearing year. The remedies come from a variety of healing arts and disciplines. Some of the remedies and techniques may be familiar to you, and others may not. I want you to feel comfortable with whatever techniques you choose, so in the next few pages I'll discuss how each type of remedy works.

What Are Body Mechanics?

Body mechanics are the way you sit, stand, walk, and lie down; they're how you move and use your muscles to perform the activities of daily living. Many of the discomforts associated with pregnancy and postpartum are caused by muscle weakness and strain. When you're pregnant, your weight rises steadily and rapidly, and then, one day the baby is born, and your weight starts dropping even faster. This relatively sudden gain and loss of weight places tremendous stress on the bones, muscles, and ligaments of your abdomen, back, hips, legs, and pelvis. As a result, you may experience aching and fatigue in your back, legs, and feet. But, you can reduce or prevent many of these problems by learning more effective ways to sit, stand, sleep, walk, and lift.

Considerations for Doing Exercises

The same physical changes mentioned above can cause other types of pain, as well as swelling, fatigue, and even poor bladder control. With the right exercises, you can give your muscles the strength and flexibility needed to adjust to the strain. For example, the right exercises will strengthen the muscles of your abdomen so that they're able to help your back support the baby's weight. Exercise also stimulates the circulation of blood through your body, resulting in decreased swelling and increased energy. These are just a few ways in which exercise can make you more comfortable while you're waiting for your baby to be born. Afterwards, exercise will make you more comfortable and will help you regain energy and muscle tone.

The changes that take place in your muscles and ligaments and bones during pregnancy and postpartum leave you more vulnerable to injury. So, while it's usually all right to participate in a well-planned and supervised prenatal or postpartal exercise class, you should never do any exercise that involves jumping or jerking, or that requires you to arch your back, as happens when you do double leg-lifts or full sit-ups. Many of the exercises in your Comfort Guide are done in slow-motion and they often involve stretching. This low-impact type of exercise will give you the best health and comfort benefits with the lowest risk of injury.

I've described each exercise step-by-step and have included simple diagrams to help you learn how to do it correctly. Before trying an exercise, read through the directions completely, following the diagrams as you read. Move slowly and easily, paying attention to how your muscles feel as they work. Don't try to push yourself farther than you comfortably can go. If an exercise calls for repetitions, start with just a few, and add one or two every three days or so, as you feel able. If the exercise requires you to hold a position for a while, start with several seconds, and gradually increase the amount of time you hold it.

If at any time an exercise seems to cause pain, stop. Review the directions and diagrams to determine if you might be doing something wrong. Think about what you felt and where. Be sure you know the difference between actual pain and the sensation of stretching a muscle that hasn't been used this way for a while. If you're not accustomed to exercise, a prolonged or overambitious stretch may feel uncomfortable. If the exercise still causes you pain, go on to something else.

Take your time building up your ability to move and stretch your body. If your muscles are sore the day after exercising, take a warm shower and follow it with a few *mild* stretches. Then omit any vigorous exercise for that day.

Remember, pain is your body's friendly warning system. It lets you know you're doing, or trying to do, something that might injure you. So, keep these two rules in mind:

❏ *Never continue an exercise that causes pain.*
❏ *Report any persistent pain to your physician or midwife.*

How to Do Proper Massage

Massage is one of the oldest and most useful comfort techniques we have. Here are a few ways massage can help:

❏ Relaxes both body and mind.
❏ Increases energy level.
❏ Reduces fatigue.
❏ Provides an increased sense of well-being.

In addition to these general benefits, certain types of massage reduce pain by stimulating your body's *endorphin system.* Endorphin is a natural pain-killer produced in the pituitary gland, just below your brain. By using the *pressure point* massage techniques you'll find in this book, you can increase your own endorphin level. In addition to helping relieve pain, certain pressure points reduce other problems, such as dizziness, tension, panic, and nausea.

Many massage techniques can be done alone, but they feel even better with a partner. Here are some guidelines to get you started.

Skin Preparation: Your hands and the skin surface to be massaged should be clean and dry. If using a stroking or kneading massage, use lotion, oil, or talc to reduce friction. *Do not use these with pressure point massage.*

Positions: If doing your own massage, find a comfortable, relaxed position that allows your arms and legs to be well-supported. If your partner is helping, you both should assume a comfortable position that allows easy access to the area to be massaged. The drawings in this book will give you some ideas.

Pressure: The amount of pressure applied depends on the comfort of the person receiving the massage. It's not necessary to cause pain. If, however, you find an area that's painful or tender or that feels fibrous or hard, you've probably uncovered a trouble spot that needs extra attention. Start with a firm, gentle touch, and gradually increase the pressure as needed.

When *giving* a massage, let the movement and pressure flow from the center of your body. Let your upper body move forward from the waist and hips each time you apply pressure. This feels better to the person you're massaging and it helps you relax so you can enjoy the massage, too.

Keeping It Safe

When using massage techniques, do not apply pressure or heat to the following:

☐ An infected area.

☐ Red or swollen skin.

☐ The inner thigh.

Certain pressure points that are not described in the Comfort Guide have been used to induce or augment labor. For this reason, it's best to avoid any point not included in this book unless you're well-trained in the use of pressure point massage during pregnancy and postpartum.

When *receiving* a massage, don't try to resist the pressure; let your body be swayed gently by the direction and rhythm of the pressure.

Breathing: Massage is always more effective if both partners breathe in rhythm to it. This reduces fatigue while helping them both relax. In some of the techniques in this book, you'll be asked to breathe in a slow, easy rhythm, similar to the pattern taught for coping with early labor. In others, you'll exhale as pressure is applied and inhale as it's released, or you'll inhale as the giver's hands move up and exhale as they move down.

When used for long periods of time, as in labor, pressure point massage sometimes loses its effectiveness. This is only temporary but, meanwhile, applications of heat or cold applied to the same area will provide a good substitute for pressure.

Importance of Good Nutrition

"You are what you eat" may never be as true for your child as it is now. The miracle of your baby's life begins with one tiny egg and one tiny sperm. It takes a lot of good nourishment for them to grow into a healthy seven- or eight-pound infant. You need the same kind of nourishment to help your body adjust to the changes and demands of pregnancy, birth, and postpartum.

As you read through the Comfort Guide, you'll discover that many of your discomforts, such as nausea, fatigue, constipation, and even bleeding gums, are often caused by nutritional deficiencies. We'll deal with specific problems later but, for now, here's what you need to eat every day if you're a pregnant or new mother:

❑ Four servings of milk products (or 1,200 milligrams of calcium).
❑ Four servings of fruits and vegetables including at least one source of vitamin A, such as leafy, green vegetables, and one source of vitamin C, such as citrus fruits, tomatoes, broccoli, or onions.
❑ Four servings of grain products (whole grains are best).
❑ Two or three servings of protein, such as chicken, fish, meat, cheese, or legumes.

In addition to the above, you also need 30-60 milligrams of iron daily. Because it's almost impossible to get this much iron from your diet, your doctor or midwife will probably prescribe an iron supplement for you.

Relaxation Techniques

The physical and emotional changes of pregnancy, birth, and postpartum cause a lot of tension and strain, which can lead to backache, headache, insomnia, fatigue, and other problems. Relaxation techniques will help you prevent or relieve these and other problems. Besides making you more comfortable now, learning to relax will give you an important tool for dealing with stress and pain throughout your life. Relaxation is a part of every major method of childbirth preparation, and it's the technique most often taught for relieving acute or chronic pain in other situations, such as surgery or injury. All the relaxation techniques have the dual purpose of relaxing and reducing pain, and any of them can be used during labor.

Throughout the Comfort Guide, I've described a variety of relaxation techniques so that you can choose those that are most effective for you. For best results, keep these suggestions in mind:

Position. Be sure your entire body, including your arms and legs, is well supported. (It's a good idea to keep several sizes of pillows handy for this purpose.)

Breathing. Start with a deep, relaxing sigh, and continue with a slow, easy breathing rhythm. Remember that exhalation is the relaxation phase of breathing, and focus on inhaling energy and exhaling tension.

Focus. Most people relax best when they concentrate on something. You might want to focus your sight on a special object, such as a baby rattle, a crucifix, or a photo or picture you really like. Or you might prefer to close your eyes and focus on an internal focal point, such as the names you've chosen for your baby or a favorite childhood memory. Throughout this book you'll discover many types of focal points, but only a few will work best for you. That's because people learn new skills, such as how to relax, according to how they relate to their world. While we all use each of our senses to experience the world, we tend to use one or two more than the others. The ones most people mention are sight, hearing, and touch. In the Comfort Guide, I'll refer to these as *sight, sound,* and *sensation.* The following questions will help you discover which of these three will give you the best relaxation cues.

❏ When you think of your favorite movie, is your strongest memory of how the actors looked or the color and style of their clothing or the scenery? When you think about the beach, do you see the sand and the sun and the sea gulls? Do you see the waves washing back and forth across the sand? If so, you're a visual, or *sight,* person. You'll relax best by focusing on the sight cues you'll find in this book.

❏ When you think of your favorite movie, is your strongest memory of the actors' voices or the music and sound effects? When you think of the beach, do you hear the roaring wind and surf or the cawing of the sea gulls? If so, you're an auditory, or *sound,* person. You'll relax best by focusing on sound cues.

❏ When you think of your favorite movie, is your strongest memory of how it made you feel? When you think of the beach, do you feel

WHAT THE EYES SHOW

You can often identify the type of relaxation cues a person needs by watching her eyes when she's talking or when she's thinking about how to answer a question. A sight person usually glances upward while thinking, a sound person usually glances to one or both sides, and a sensation person usually glances downward.

Soothing Sounds

No matter what type of cues you prefer, it may help to include some sort of auditory cue, such as music, to block out the sounds of your environment. (This is especially important in a hospital labor area—one of the busiest and noisiest parts of a hospital.) After trying dozens of sounds in my classes, the ones I'd recommend you try are your partner's voice and these two recordings:

❏ "Environments: Totally New Concepts in Sound, Disc 4—The Ultimate Thunderstorm." There's something about a thunderstorm that reminds many people of their childhood, when they climbed into bed, pulled the sheets up high, and rested safely while the rain and thunder played outside their window. Play this recording softly to provide an unobtrusive background noise that covers other, more distracting noises.

❏ "Jonathan Livingston Seagull," by Neil Diamond. The slower portions of this recording are ideal for learning relaxation and for relaxing during labor. Many couples find that the faster portions work well for advanced labor, when the work requires an already-tired woman to stay awake and alert in order to keep up with the pace and strength of contractions.

the heat of the sun, the gentle motion of the breeze on your skin, or the soft, warm sand under your feet? If so, you're a kinesthetic, or *sensation*, person. You'll relax best by focusing on sensation cues.

When to Use Cold or Heat Therapy

COLD

Apply cold to:

- ❑ Reduce swelling or pain due to an injury that's no more than an hour old.
- ❑ Reduce swelling or pain caused by too much blood flow to an area.
- ❑ Numb a painful area, such as an aching back.
- ❑ Substitute for pressure if a pressure point massage technique becomes temporarily ineffective due to prolonged use.

HEAT

Apply heat to:

- ❑ Reduce swelling or pain due to an injury that's more than an hour old.
- ❑ Relax and soothe tired or sore muscles.
- ❑ Increase blood flow to an area.
- ❑ Reduce prolonged pain in a muscle or bone.
- ❑ Substitute for pressure if a pressure point massage technique becomes temporarily ineffective due to prolonged use.

Healing With Herbal Therapy

Many cultures, including my husband's own Mexican culture, have used herbs for centuries to heal the body and to promote health. Unfortunately, there has been little scientific research on herbs, so most of the information we have comes from herbalists, curanderos, and other practitioners who have handed down their remedies from generation to generation. My own experience with herbs is limited to what my mother-in-law taught me as I saw my husband and children through colds, colic, diarrhea, stomach-aches, headaches, and a dozen other problems that are simply a part of being human.

Keep in mind that herbs were our first medicines and, while they can have a healing effect, some of them may also cause side effects. In researching herbs for this book, I found no evidence of danger among those listed, except for a rare and dangerous allergic reaction to chamomile (manzanilla). If you have a history of multiple allergies or if you're allergic to ragweed, it would be wise to avoid this herb.

Labor Tips

Certain discomforts, such as back pain or nausea, can happen not only during pregnancy, but during labor, too. You'll find special tips to help you deal with these problems under the appropriate heading in the prenatal section of the Comfort Guide. For example, if you want to know how to deal with the pain of back labor, look up "Backache" in the prenatal section of the book, and then keep your eyes open for the "Labor Tips" sign with the hand symbol.

Special Situations

All the discomforts covered in this Comfort Guide are the result of the normal changes of pregnancy. But, sometimes the normal demands of pregnancy create an abnormal response, such as high blood pressure, diabetes, bleeding, or preeclampsia (toxemia). These special situations that occur in a small percentage of women are more than discomforts—they're complications. Unlike other changes of pregnancy, you can't handle these situations by yourself, and you shouldn't try.

Because complications must be dealt with by you and your birth attendant, and because there are still unsettled controversies about how to treat most of these situations, we won't deal with them in this book. Throughout the Comfort Guide, you'll find warnings to notify your birth attendant if you experience certain symptoms that indicate a possible complication. Located at the beginning of the prenatal section and the postpartum section you'll also find charts explaining how you can determine whether what you're experiencing is a normal discomfort or the warning sign of a possible problem. Please take these warnings seriously.

PART ONE

PREGNANCY

DISCOMFORTS AND DANGER SIGNS OF PREGNANCY

With all the changes in your body, you may have difficulty knowing if a discomfort you feel is a natural part of pregnancy or a sign of a problem. This chart describes the discomforts and danger signs that are most often confused and shows how to tell the difference. Because no two pregnancies are alike, your doctor's advice may vary from theses suggestions. Please discuss with your doctor and your childbirth educator any measures you may take or any question you have.

PROBLEM	ACTION	CAUSE
SWELLING Feet and ankles swell after prolonged sitting or standing.	Lie on left side with feet elevated for 15 to 30 minutes. *Prevention:* Exercise regularly. Drink eight glasses of water daily. Avoid prolonged standing or sitting.	Normal increase in fluid and blood volume. Uterine pressure on blood vessels in legs.
Swelling isn't better after elevating feet for 30 minutes.	NOTIFY YOUR BIRTH ATTENDANT.	May signal excess fluid retention or a more serious condition.
Both hands are swollen.	NOTIFY YOUR BIRTH ATTENDANT.	May signal preeclampsia or high blood pressure.
One hand swells after you've slept on that side of body.	Raise hand over head, wiggling fingers to aid circulation.	Sleep position interfered with blood flow in arm.
Face and/or eyes are puffy or swollen.	NOTIFY YOUR BIRTH ATTENDANT.	May signal preeclampsia or high blood pressure.
LEG PAIN Painful area is hot, red, or swollen.	NOTIFY YOUR BIRTH ATTENDANT.	May indicate blood clot.
Sharp cramp in calf (charley horse).	Sit with leg straight, foot flexed. Gently reach toward foot.	Cause not definite; may be due to too much or too little calcium.
VAGINAL DISCHARGE Thin mucus discharge; pale yellow or colorless.	Ask if doctor wants to be notified of changes.	Normal hormonal changes. (Increase may indicate approaching labor.)
Bloody discharge.	NOTIFY YOUR BIRTH ATTENDANT.	May signal start of labor or may signal serious problem with placenta.
Thin, watery discharge.	NOTIFY YOUR BIRTH ATTENDANT.	May indicate amniotic sac has broken.
ABDOMINAL DISCOMFORT Sharp pain in side or groin, lasting less than two minutes.	Bend at waist, toward the pain; relax, and breathe slowly. *Prevention:* Avoid rapid changes of position.	Spasm of ligament holding uterus to pelvis.
Pain accompanied by rigid abdomen, nausea or vomiting, or dizziness; or pain lasting more than two minutes.	NOTIFY YOUR BIRTH ATTENDANT IMMEDIATELY.	May indicate ememgency with placenta or uterus.
Intermittent cramping and/or abdominal tightening.	NOTIFY YOUR BIRTH ATTENDANT IF SYMPTOMS OCCUR MORE THAN SIX TIMES IN AN HOUR.	May be labor contractions.

OTHER DANGER SIGNS:
• persistent vomiting
• persistent headaches
• visual disturbances
• major decrease in urine
• major decrease in fetal movement
NOTIFY YOUR BIRTH ATTENDANT.

Abdominal Pressure

"The bigger the baby gets, the more uncomfortable my stomach gets. You know what I'm talking about, don't you? That feeling that your maternity pants are made wrong . . . that the stretch panel stops too soon."

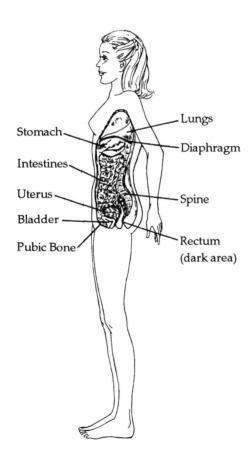

Stomach

Intestines

Uterus

Bladder

Pubic Bone

Lungs

Diaphragm

Spine

Rectum
(dark area)

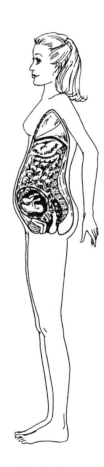

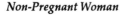

Non-Pregnant Woman

Four Months Pregnant

As your pregnancy progresses, you'll probably feel pressure or pulling in your lower abdomen. This uncomfortable sensation is caused by the increasing weight of your uterus, along with the placenta, the amniotic fluid, and, of course, your baby.

As your abdomen begins to bulge over the front part of your hipbone (the *pubic bone*), other people start to notice. In other words, you begin to "show." This happens about the fourth month if you're expecting your first baby, and about the third month if you already have had children. For a little while, your hips may continue to support the extra weight. But, as your baby keeps growing, your abdomen protrudes past the pubic bone, where gravity takes over, pulling downward on the weight. This means the skin, muscles, and nerves are sandwiched between the pubic bone and the baby. This leaves your lower abdomen feeling both overstretched and cramped for space, all at the same time.

If this isn't your first baby, you may notice more abdominal pressure and discomfort than with your other babies, and you may feel it

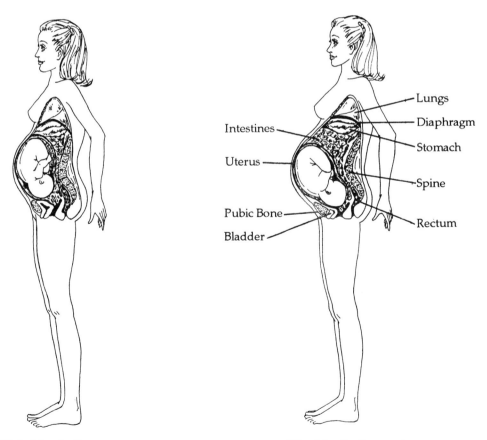

Eight Months Pregnant   *Nine Months Pregnant*

sooner. But don't worry—this doesn't necessarily mean that you made a mistake about the date of conception and that your baby is due sooner than you thought. Instead, this earlier and increased discomfort is probably due to the fact that your previous pregnancies left your muscles weakened and unable to support your abdomen as well as before. As a result, you'll tend to carry the baby lower and farther out, which, unfortunately, increases the feelings of abdominal pressure and pulling.

COMFORT

What to Do

☐ Use exercises and positions that take the weight of the baby off your lower abdomen:

- Bridge (page 7).
- Knee-Chest (page 7).

☐ Use exercises that strengthen your abdominal muscles:

- Pelvic Tilt (page 10).
- Buttocks Curl (page 11).
- Curl-Ups (page 12).

Tips for Choosing Abdominal Exercises

In choosing exercises for the abdominal area, keep these tips in mind:

☐ To prevent straining your back or abdomen, keep your knees bent when lying on your back and slightly bent when standing.

☐ Keep all movements smooth and gradual, without jerking. If you need to jerk or grunt to finish a movement, stop.

☐ Avoid double leg-lifts and full sit-ups during pregnancy. (A half sit-up is often more beneficial and always safer than a full sit-up.)

EXERCISE TECHNIQUES

BRIDGE

Benefits: Takes the weight of the baby off your abdomen, eases backache and back tension, and enhances circulation.

1. Lie on your back with your knees bent and your feet flat on the floor and close to your buttocks.
2. Press your waist to the floor, using your hips and thighs to lift your tailbone a few inches off the floor.
3. Keep going, lifting your lower spine just a few inches off the floor.
4. Continue to lift your spine, raising one bone at a time.
5. When you're as high as you can go, try to hold the position for five seconds before lowering your spine, just as slowly as you raised it, one bone at a time.

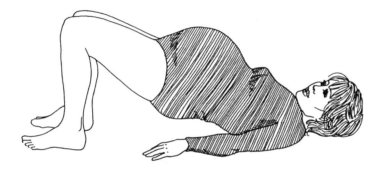

The Bridge

KNEE-CHEST

Benefits: Takes the weight of the baby off your lower abdomen; and helps improve circulation and relieve gas, constipation, and backaches.

1. Start on your hands and knees with a large cushion in front of you. (See figure on page 8.)
2. Place your hands underneath the cushion.
3. Slowly drop your elbows to the floor (or bed), resting your head and chest on the cushion.
4. Move your knees forward a bit until your back feels rounded and comfortable.
5. Hold the position for five or ten seconds. As you get used to the Knee-Chest, try to hold it longer. Focus on relaxing your body as you rest in this position.

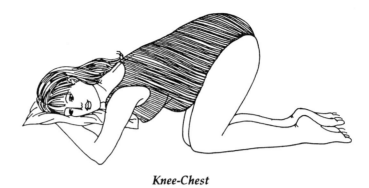

Knee-Chest

To get out of the Knee-Chest:

1. Push against your hands, stretching your arms out straight into a prayer posture.
2. Slowly pull out of the position, uncurling your spine one bone at a time until you're sitting on your knees.

Comments: The Knee-Chest should be done very slowly. At first, it may feel like the blood is rushing to your head, and you may not feel comfortable in this position for more than a few seconds. But as you practice, you'll gradually be able to hold the position longer and you'll get more benefit from it. (I've always found it curious that so many women tell me this position actually gets more comfortable the farther along they go in their pregnancy.)

(*See also* Abdominal Weakness, page 8; Backache, page 15; and Pelvic Pressure, page 96.)

Abdominal Weakness

During pregnancy, there's a lot of pressure and strain on your abdominal muscles, and this often means backaches and abdominal discomforts, as well as stretch marks. With the right exercises, you can strengthen these muscles and reduce or eliminate these problems.

As you can see in the figure on page 10, your abdominal wall is made up of several sets of muscles. The diagonal, or *oblique,* muscles run down the side of your abdomen. They help support the weight of your uterus and other organs, and they give definition to your waistline. The vertical, or *recti,* muscles run down the front of your abdomen and meet in the middle. These muscles are like two strong, protective sheets over many of your vital organs, as well as over your growing child. Both sets of abdominal muscles do a lot of stretching as your baby grows, but there are several steps you can take to strengthen them so that they will offer you a maximum of protection and support.

Preventing the Separation of Abdominal Muscles

The recti muscles come together at the center of our abdomen, similar to the fabric panels of a tight shirt that has a seam running down the front. If the seam receives too much stress, it may give way, separating at its weakest point. The same thing can happen to your abdominal muscles, allowing the uterus to protrude between them. This separation, called *diastasis recti*, can happen gradually as the muscles fail to support the growing uterus, or it can happen suddenly during strenuous activity. A common cause of diastasis is prolonged straining during the pushing phase of childbirth, but it can also happen if you lift something heavy or if you attempt an exercise for which you're not prepared. The separation may be so slight that it's barely noticeable, or so great that the uterus starts to bulge through the opening. (If this happens, your doctor may say you have a *hernia*. This just means that something is protruding through the muscle wall.)

If the muscles do separate, they'll leave your abdomen even weaker, and this can mean more backaches, difficulty in pushing, and slower recovery of muscle tone after the birth. If the problem isn't corrected, it will probably get worse in future pregnancies.

In order to protect yourself from this problem, it's important to determine whether you already have any extra abdominal weakness *before* you start exercising. If so, you'll need to do the exercises differently. Here's how to test the strength of your abdominal wall:

1. Lie on your back with your knees bent and arms stretched to the front.
2. Slowly lift your head and shoulders until they clear the floor by about eight inches. If the recti muscles have separated, you'll probably see a soft, vertical bulge in the center of your abdomen.

If you're not showing yet, or if you don't see a bulge when you lift your head, try this test:

1. Place the fingertips of one hand on the midline of your abdomen and feel for two vertical ridges of muscle on either side.
2. With your fingers in place, slowly lift your head and shoulders as before. If you feel a soft space about an inch wide, running between the two recti muscles, you may have a separation.

If you have a separation, you should avoid doing double leg-raises, sit-ups, or any other exercise that puts extra strain on the recti muscles. Two exercises that can help are the Kneeling Pelvic Tilt (page 19) and the Buttocks Curl (page 11). When you do abdominal exercises, cross your arms over your abdomen to brace your sides. This will give extra support to your abdomen.

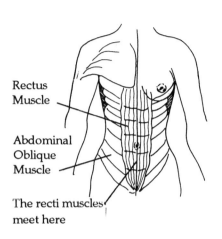

Rectus
Muscle

Abdominal
Oblique
Muscle

The recti muscles
meet here

Abdominal Muscles

PREVENTION

What to Do

❑ Use the following exercises:

- Pelvic Tilt (described below). (Develop the habit of maintaining a pelvic tilt as much as possible when you walk, stand, or sit.)
- Side Slide (page 11).
- Buttocks Curl (page 11).
- Curl-Ups (page 12).

What to Avoid

❑ Avoid exercises that require you to lift both legs at the same time.

❑ Avoid full sit-ups. (For a safe way to do sit-ups, see the directions for Curl-Ups, page 12.)

COMFORT

What to Do

❑ Use the exercises listed under "Prevention."

❑ When lifting something from below waist level, keep your back straight and bend your knees as you pick it up. Then tighten your abdomen and push yourself up with your legs.

What to Avoid

❑ Avoid lifting heavy objects.

❑ See Prevention tips, "What to Avoid," above.

EXERCISE TECHNIQUES

PELVIC TILT

Benefits: Strengthens abdominal muscles and eases lower back pain.

1. Sit or stand in a comfortable position.
2. Inhale and relax.
3. Exhale and tighten your abdominal muscles while tilting your hips upward toward your tummy, as though trying to lift your baby to your chest.
4. Hold for a count of five.

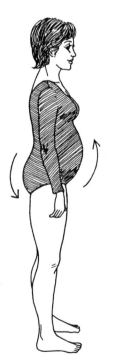

Standing Pelvic Tilt

5. Inhale and release.
6. Repeat three times.
7. When you feel comfortable with the exercise, gradually increase the number of repetitions and the length of time you hold your muscles tight.

SIDE SLIDE

Benefits: Strengthens oblique (diagonal) abdominal muscles and improves flexibility.

1. Stand with your feet about twelve to eighteen inches apart, your arms at your sides.
2. Inhale and relax.
3. Exhale and bend to the right at the waist, sliding your right arm down the side of your leg as far as you comfortably can.
4. Inhale, while holding the position for a slow count of three.
5. Exhale, using your oblique waistline muscles to pull yourself back up to the starting position.
6. Repeat on left side.
7. Try to do at least three repetitions a day, gradually increasing the length of time you hold the stretch.

   Comments: Be sure to stretch to the side, with your head and torso facing forward; try to not let your upper body twist to the side. For an added benefit, use the opposite arm to reach over your head while you are bending.

BUTTOCKS CURL

Benefits: Strengthens abdominal muscles and eases lower back pain.

1. Lie on your back, bending your knees up over your abdomen so that your feet are off the floor.
2. Inhale as you relax for a moment in this position.
3. Exhale, tightening your belly as you press your waist to the floor. (This action is the same as the Pelvic Tilt, and it should lift your buttocks slightly off the floor.)
4. Hold for a count of three, inhaling and exhaling as needed.
5. Inhale and release.
6. Repeat five times. As you feel more comfortable with this exercise, try to gradually lengthen the count, and increase the number of repetitions.

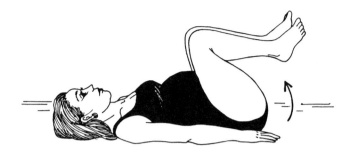

Buttocks Curl

Comments: Do the Buttocks Curl slowly and deliberately, without jerking or bouncing. Focus on using your abdomen, not your hips, to pull your baby toward your chest.

If your abdominal muscles are already well-toned and you'd like more of a challenge, try this next exercise:

CURL-UPS

Benefits: Strengthens abdominal muscles.

1. Lie on your back with your knees bent and arms to the side.
2. Inhale and relax.
3. Exhale slowly, raising your head and then your shoulders off the floor and keeping your arms stretched in front of you.
4. Continue exhaling as you gradually lift your upper body as far as you can comfortably go, *but no farther* than a semi-sitting position.
5. If you feel you must jerk or grunt in order to go any further, stop and move on to the next step.
6. Inhale as you slowly lower your upper body to the floor.

Comments: Think of your spinal bones as a string of pearls lying on

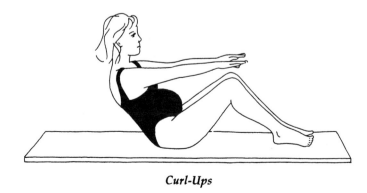

Curl-Ups

the floor. Now, lift the string off the floor, one pearl at a time, and then lower it one pearl at a time.

(*See also* Abdominal Pressure, page 4; Abdominal Weakness, post-partal, page 120; and Backache, prenatal, page 15.)

Anemia

Like most expectant moms, you may tire more easily now than before you were pregnant. This feeling of chronic fatigue is caused by a variety of factors, such as hormonal changes, weight gain, and anemia. While you can't do much about the hormonal changes or weight gain, you can get a great deal of relief if you take care of the anemia.

Someone who has anemia, or who is *anemic,* has fewer red blood cells than are needed. Without enough red cells, the blood can't clot. This means you could experience excessive bleeding if you injure yourself, and that you and your baby are more prone to bleeding during or after the birth. Red blood cells are also important because they contain *hemoglobin,* which carries oxygen from your lungs all through your body. So, if you're anemic, your muscles and bones, as well as your brain and other organs, aren't getting enough oxygen to keep them functioning at their best. And your baby may not be getting enough oxygen to keep her growing and developing at her best.

Anemia sometimes results from excessive bleeding during an operation or following an injury or miscarriage. But the most common cause of anemia is a diet low in iron, the mineral that helps your body make hemoglobin. As an expectant mother, you naturally need more iron than other women because it takes extra red blood cells to meet the in-

---

Signs of Anemia

Let your birth attendant know if you're experiencing any of these symptoms:

- ❑ Weakness.
- ❑ Fatigue.
- ❑ Shortness of breath.
- ❑ Pale skin.
- ❑ Palpitations (a feeling that your heart is beating faster and harder than usual).

About Anemia

WHAT ABOUT VITAMIN SUPPLEMENTS?

Even with a well-balanced diet, it's almost impossible to get enough iron from your daily food intake, so most physicians prescribe iron supplements for their pregnant patients. The iron may be prescribed as an individual supplement, or as part of a multiple vitamins-and-minerals supplement. A prescription is not required for most vitamins and minerals, so you can buy an over-the-counter preparation if you like. But be careful that you don't take more than the pregnancy recommended daily allowance (RDA). This is especially important with fat-soluble vitamins, such as A, D, and E, which are stored in your body and may build up to levels that are harmful to you or your baby.

If you still develop anemia, your doctor may give you larger doses of oral iron. If your condition calls for stronger measures, or if you cannot take iron by mouth, he may give it to you through injections. Iron can upset your stomach or cause diarrhea, so be sure to take the liquid or tablets right after a meal. If this doesn't help, ask your doctor or pharmacist for a different form of iron, one that is easier on the stomach.

FACT OR FICTION?

If you have a persistent craving for ice, it means you're anemic. The experts have argued over this belief for decades, and they still don't agree. But, about 25 percent of those expectant mothers who are anemic do report eating large amounts of ice or nonfood substances, such as laundry starch. While eating ice isn't harmful, eating large quantities of starch or any other nonfood item can be. In fact, it can make the anemia worse because you're filling up on things that give no nourishment to you or your baby. So, if you experience this type of craving, let your birth attendant know so she can check you for anemia.

Drinking red wine will thicken the blood. This is completely false, and it could also be dangerous for your baby. We know that large amounts of alcohol can cause your baby to develop *Fetal Alcohol Syndrome*, a condition that involves both mental and physical abnormalities. Unfortunately, no one has been able to determine if there is a safe level of consumption and, if so, what it is. So, right now, the safest way to handle alcohol is to avoid it completely until after your baby is born. If you'll be breastfeeding her, wait until after she's weaned before you resume drinking alcohol.

creased demands that pregnancy places on your body. In fact, you need about 30-60 milligrams of iron each day. This is about two to four times the amount required by other women, and about three to six times that required by men.

PREVENTION

What to Do

❑ Eat iron-rich foods from animal sources, such as liver, tongue, heart, and other organ or lean meats, oysters, clams, and eggs. (Animal products are the best dietary source of iron.)

- ❏ For animal products lower in cholesterol and fat, choose fish or chicken.
- ❏ For vegetarian sources, choose beans, peas, whole grains, prunes, raisins, leafy green vegetables, and black strap molasses. (Some leafy greens contain a substance that makes it difficult for your body to absorb iron, so don't depend on these alone.)
- ❏ Make sure your diet includes enough calcium and vitamin C, both of which increase the body's ability to absorb iron. Calcium is found in milk products, and vitamin C is found in citrus fruits, tomatoes, potatoes, broccoli, and onions. Cook some of your meals in cast-iron pots and pans. Some foods absorb the iron as they cook. (There is controversy over whether this type of iron can be absorbed and used by the body.)
- ❏ Focus on balance in all parts of your diet because, in addition to iron, a number of other nutrients are involved in making hemoglobin. Every day, eat several servings each of fresh fruits and vegetables, whole grains, and milk products, as well as iron-rich foods.
- ❏ Take a daily vitamin-mineral supplement containing iron.

COMFORT

What to Do

- ❏ Follow dietary tips listed under "Prevention."
- ❏ Try to arrange your schedule so that you sleep at least eight hours a night and rest several times a day.
- ❏ Exercise regularly, focusing on activities that improve circulation, such as walking, swimming, or stationary bicycling.

What to Avoid

- ❏ Avoid overexertion.

Backache

"I don't know which I hate worse—the backache or the weight gain."

"What's the worst thing? Definitely the backache. I rub her back every night to help her get to sleep, but she still hurts when she wakes up in the morning."

Backache is one of the most common discomforts of pregnancy. By the seventh month, most women are having problems with lower back pain, and some have pain in the upper back, too. Here's why: In early pregnancy your baby rests on your hipbones, which are quite strong and can support a lot of weight. But, as your baby grows, the weight pushes forward, past your pubic bone. When this happens, gravity starts to pull the weight forward and downward, forcing your back muscles to arch. It's this constant muscular tension that makes your lower back hurt.

As your baby continues to grow, your abdominal organs are crowded up into the chest area where they put pressure on your ribs, pushing them outward and straining your rib cage. This places the muscles between the ribs in a state of constant tension, leaving them aching and tired. Besides being an uncomfortable nuisance, such persistent aching can leave you physically and emotionally exhausted.

MAKING PREVENTION A HABIT

Because many of the routine activities you perform every day can lead to backaches, it's a good idea to try to be more aware of *how* you perform these tasks and how they affect your back. For example, when driving, do you feel a tightness in your lower back? If you do, or if you're not sure, do a Pelvic Tilt and then relax your spine. (To do a Pelvic Tilt while sitting, simply tilt your hips upward and forward as though trying to lift your baby to your chest. This should leave your back slightly rounded.) After doing this, your back should feel more relaxed. Now, what about your shoulders? Lift and then drop them, dropping all the tension, too. And now your lower jaw—release the tension, letting the jaw drop slightly to relax your neck muscles. (Yes, you can do this and still keep your mouth closed!) Being more aware of how you use your body helps prevent many of the aches and pains that bother you. It's also great practice for labor, when you'll want to reduce pain or discomfort by relaxing the rest of your body while your uterus works.

PREVENTION

What to Do

☐ Stand, sit, and sleep using positions that relax and protect your back. To do this, remember that when one or both of your hips are flexed, your back muscles can relax. The Pelvic Tilt (page 10) does this, but you can't go around all day Pelvic Tilting, so try these:

- *Standing.* Try to avoid prolonged standing, but, if you have to do it, rest one foot on a box or stool. If you're in a grocery line, rest your foot on the lower rack of the grocery cart. Working in the kitchen, open the cabinet door under the sink and rest your foot on the lower shelf.

- *Sitting.* Try to avoid sitting in one position for more than half an hour. To further ease the strain on your back, keep a small box or footstool or a thick telephone book nearby and occasionally rest one or both feet on it.

- *Sleeping.* Use pillows to keep one or both hips slightly flexed. If you sleep on your back (not a great idea after the fourth month of pregnancy) put a small pillow under your thighs. If you sleep on your side, bend your knees and put a pillow between them. And if you *wish* you could still sleep on your stomach, here's how I worked it out when I was pregnant—put several pillows under your hips and one or two under your head and chest, so that you make a nest for your tummy. Now, snuggle down, get comfy, and sweet dreams!

❑ Use your legs and abdominal muscles when lifting something from below waist level—keep your back straight and bend your knees to reach the object, then tighten your abdomen and push yourself up with your legs.

❑ To prevent a lower backache, strengthen your abdominal muscles so they can hold your baby in closer to your body and reduce the arch in your spine. Try these exercises:

- Kneeling Pelvic Tilt (page 19).
- Buttocks Curl (page 11).
- Curl-Ups (page 12).
- Knee-Chest (page 7).

❑ To prevent an upper backache, focus on releasing the tension from your shoulders, neck, and jaw throughout the day. A quick way to do this is to tighten these muscles just a bit, and then to let go. (Notice that when you let go of your jaw and shoulders, they drop downward, into a relaxed position. Try to keep them in this relaxed, downward position as much as possible.)

What to Avoid

❑ Avoid lifting heavy objects.

❑ Avoid exercises and activities that require you to lift both legs at the same time or to arch your back.

COMFORT

What to Do

❑ Stand, sit, and sleep in the preventive positions described above.

❑ Do exercises for lower backache listed under prevention tips, "What to Do," above.

❑ Do exercises to help relieve upper backache:

- Forward Bend (page 20).
- Shoulder Circles (page 21).

❑ Try these massages:

- Lower Back Massage (page 21).
- Shoulder Massage (page 22).
- Total Back Massage (page 23).

❑ Apply heat or cold to the painful area. Try a heating pad or hot-

ROCKING AWAY THE PAIN

When I was expecting my second child, I had problems with lower back pain. Although I hadn't yet learned about exercise and massage techniques, I frequently found temporary relief by rocking in my old-fashioned, curved-back rocker. Several times a day I'd put my two-year-old son, Daniel, in my lap and start rocking. The aching usually eased after the first few minutes, and Daniel and I got in a little extra "together time."

water bottle, or try a warm bath or shower if muscular tension is causing your pain, or if you want an all-over relaxing effect. For more persistent pain or pain caused by the baby's position against the spine, cold is often more effective. The chemical ice packs sold in sporting goods stores may work better than an ice bag or washcloth filled with ice cubes because the chemical pack remains hard, allowing you to apply both cold and pressure at the same time.

What to Avoid

❑ Avoid taking any pain medication without your birth attendant's okay.

❑ Avoid taking aspirin or ibuprofen.

LABOR TIPS

Upper Back Pain

If pain is in the upper back, try the following techniques:

❑ Apply pressure, heat, or cold to the shoulder pressure points to relieve upper back pain or stiffness during labor.

❑ Use the shoulder points to detect and relieve tension or fatigue throughout the body. Many couples find it helpful if the labor coach occasionally places his hands on his partner's shoulder points during a contraction. If tension or fatigue is present, the points will probably tighten or harden as the contraction continues.

Lower Back Pain

If pain is in the lower back, try the following techniques:

❑ Use the lower back points for lower back pain, tension, or fatigue. As labor progresses, your baby's position will change and the location of the pain may change, too. Even if the spinal pressure points aren't in the same place as your pain, they can help, so give them a try.

❑ For back pain during late labor, apply firm pressure, heat, or cold to points located on either side of the tailbone. They start just below the top ridge of your hipbone and are located in the grooves of the tailbone. Because your backbone is wider here, the grooves are a little harder to find. Fortunately, most people have a terrific landmark—the two little dimples, or indentations, just above the buttocks are about the same distance apart as the spinal grooves in the tailbone.

(If you can't see the dimples in the back, you can still find the points by remembering that this part of your spine is about as wide as your hand when measured from the outer edge of the first finger to the outer edge of the little finger. Be sure to measure *your* hand to locate the points on *your* back and *your partner's* hand to locate those on *his* back.)

Back Labor

In many labors, the pain or discomfort is felt mostly in the abdomen, and it comes and goes with each contraction. In *back labor*, which occurs in about 30 percent of labors, the pain is felt mostly in the back, and it remains strong and constant, increasing with contractions, but never quite disappearing between them. The back pain comes from the pressure of the baby's head on the mother's lower spine. Walking during labor can help relieve the back pain and will also help the labor progress at a good pace. Here's how you can combine walking and massage in a special technique called the Slow Dance:

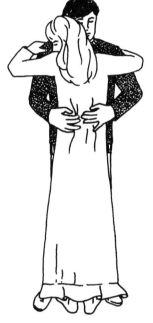

Slow Dance

1. Between contractions stroll slowly, arm in arm, in the room or hallway.
2. As a contraction begins, turn and face your partner as if you were about to do a slow dance. Put your arms around his neck and rest your head and the weight of your upper body on his shoulder or chest.
3. Meanwhile, your partner puts his arms around your waist and uses his fingers to apply firm, circular pressure to the points on your lower back.

Comments: Couples who've used the Slow Dance technique say it's even more effective and relaxing when they gently sway side to side in rhythm with their favorite slow music.

EXERCISE TECHNIQUES

KNEELING PELVIC TILT

Benefits: Eases back pain and strengthens abdominal muscles.

1. Start on your hands and knees, with your back relaxed, not arched.
2. Inhale and relax a moment.
3. Exhale and pull in your buttocks. (Pretend you're a puppy, tucking in your tail.)
4. Hold for a count of three.
5. Inhale and relax.

6. Repeat five times. Gradually increase the number of repetitions and the length of time you hold the tilt.

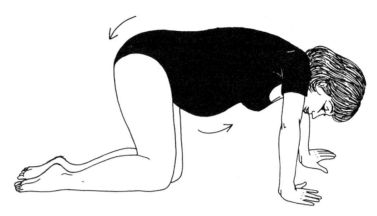

Kneeling Pelvic Tilt

FORWARD BEND

Benefits: Eases back pain by stretching the entire spine, reduces tension and fatigue, and increases energy.

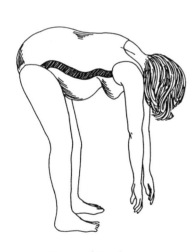

Forward Bend

1. Stand with your feet about twelve to eighteen inches apart and your knees slightly bent. *(Do not keep your legs straight; do not lock your knees.)*
2. Bend forward at the waist, reaching your hands toward the floor and letting your upper body sag forward, like an inflatable doll slowly losing its air.
3. Continue bending as far as you comfortably can. (To protect your back and knees, keep your knees bent slightly and spread your legs as much as needed for comfort.)
4. Still bending from the waist, sway your torso from side to side, making a wide arc with your hands. Be sure to keep these movements loose and easy.
5. Continue to sway until your back feels more relaxed.
6. To come out of this position, slowly uncurl your spine, one backbone at a time, so that the last thing up is your shoulders. (This final step is important. Never come up from a forward bend with your back straight. This puts too much weight on your lower spine and may hurt your back.)

SHOULDER CIRCLES

Benefits: Eases upper backache, relieves stiffness or aching in the shoulders, and reduces tension and fatigue.

1. Shrug both shoulders and release.
2. Lift both shoulders and circle them toward your back, then down, and then toward the front.
3. After several full circles, finish with one big sigh as you shrug and then drop your shoulders straight down. (As you do this exercise, feel how your shoulder blades actually massage your upper back.)

Comments: You can do this exercise almost anywhere—at your desk, in your car, standing in line at the store. You'll get the most relief if you circle your shoulders toward your back, inhaling as they move up and exhaling as they move down.

"During late labor, when I was exhausted and ready to quit, my husband started massaging my back. All at once, I felt his love and energy flow into my body, giving me the strength to keep going."

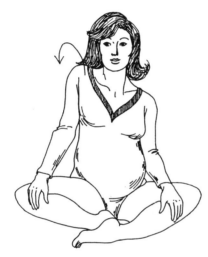

Shoulder Circles

MASSAGE TECHNIQUES

LOWER BACK MASSAGE

Benefits: Relieves pain and tension in lower back, and reduces fatigue.

1. Place your hands on your waist, with the fingers pointing toward the spine.
2. Slide your hands toward the center of your back until the longest fingers reach the two grooves on either side of your spine. That's where these two special pressure points are (see figure, right).
3. Use your thumbs, fingers, or fists to apply firm, steady pressure or to massage these pressure points in a small, circular pattern.
4. If you prefer stronger pressure, ask your partner to use the heels of his hands for this massage. If no partner is available, lie on your bed in a semi-sitting position and fold your hands into fists and use your knuckles to apply strong, steady pressure.

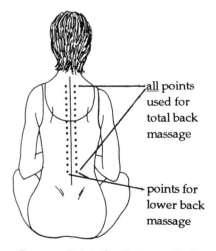

all points used for total back massage

points for lower back massage

Pressure Points for the Lower Back Massage and Total Back Massage

SHOULDER MASSAGE

Benefits: Reduces pain and tension in neck, shoulders, and upper back; can also relieve headache and reduce fatigue.

1. Place your right hand on your left shoulder so that the thumb lies alongside your neck. (See point A on figure "Pressure Points for Shoulder Massage." Reverse procedure to locate right shoulder point.)
2. Move your fingers forward just a little, toward the top of your shoulder, until you reach a place where the muscle is slightly raised or rounded.

    (If you're not sure you've found the right spot, you can check it by placing your fingers over your left breast and moving them in a direct line from the nipple up to the shoulder, stopping just behind the top of the shoulder.)

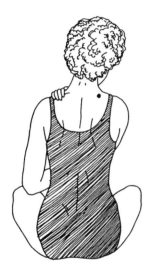

*Pressure Points for
Shoulder Massage*

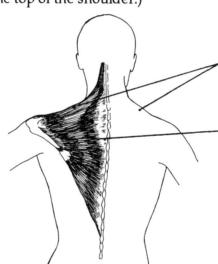

*Pressure Points for Shoulder Massage,
Located on the Trapezius Muscle*

Try these three massage techniques on the shoulder points:

1. *Pressure:* Use a firm, circular pattern, gently moving the skin over the bone.
    Breathing: Inhale and exhale in a slow, relaxed rhythm.
2. *Pressure:* Apply firm, intermittent pressure, holding it for a slow count of four, and releasing for a slow count of four. Continue for one minute or longer. (Be sure to maintain skin-to-skin contact with your partner. Release the pressure, but not the touch.)
    Breathing: Exhale as pressure is applied, and inhale as it's released. (Let your partner know if he's pressing too quickly or too slowly for you to breathe comfortably.)

3. For relief from backache, headache, tension, and fatigue, you can't beat this massage:

    Pressure: Beginning at the shoulder points, use your fingers to apply firm, circular pressure for ten seconds.

    Next, gently slide your fingers up toward the neck, so that they are just above the shoulder points, and repeat the firm, circular pressure for ten seconds.

    Continue moving up the side of the neck, each time gently sliding your fingers just above the previous points. As you move onto the neck, your fingers should be just outside the ridges of muscle that lie on either side of your spine.

    When you reach the lower edge of the skull bone, use all your fingers to press up toward the bone and apply ten seconds of firm, circular massage.

    For further relaxation, continue the massage, moving along the hairline until you reach the temples.

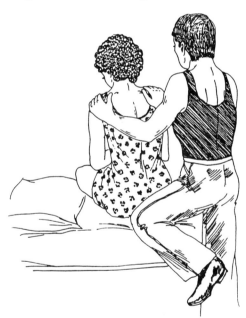

Shoulder Massage by Partner During Labor

TOTAL BACK MASSAGE

Benefits: Reduces pain in back, shoulders, and neck, and relaxes full body.

Pressure points along either side of your spine help relieve backache, tension, and fatigue. To find them, place your fingers or thumbs on either side of your spine. You should feel a slight indentation, or groove, running lengthwise on either side of the backbone. One set of pressure points is located along each groove. You can spend a lot of time learning just where each point is, but an easier and more relaxing way to stimulate these and other back points is with an old-fashioned back rub. You'll need a partner for this one. Here's what he should do:

1. Help your partner to sit forward and to use pillows to support her upper body and arms.
2. Warm a liberal amount of lotion in your hands, and then place your hands so that the heels rest on the upper buttocks and the thumbs rest on the lower back points (see figure on page 21 for lower back points).
3. Slowly and firmly push your hands up toward her neck, keeping your thumbs in or near the spinal grooves.
4. When you reach the neck, slide your hands out until the fingers rest on the shoulder points, where you'll give a brief, kneading massage.
5. Continue by pulling your hands out along the shoulder blades and down the middle of each side of her back.
6. When you reach the lower back, slide your hands inward to the starting position and begin again.
7. Breathing for this massage is: inhale as the hands move up the back, exhale as they move down. Use a slow, relaxed breathing pattern and match the movement to it.

Comments: One mother said this massage felt as though her husband were drawing a large heart on her back.

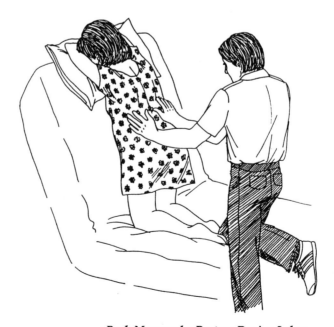

Back Massage by Partner During Labor

Balance Disturbances

Have you noticed that it's easier to lose your balance now than before you got pregnant? This is because your center of gravity has changed. If you gain weight when you're not pregnant, you gain it slowly and all over your body. But, now that you're pregnant, the weight comes on fast, and most of it is located right in the front center of your body. No wonder you lose your footing more easily now!

Unfortunately, the problem may worsen later in pregnancy when your body releases a hormone called *relaxin*. Its function is to soften your cervix so that it can open in labor, and to relax the cartilage between your hipbones so that they spread slightly, making more room for the baby.

The problem is that relaxin can also affect the cartilage in other parts of your body. Some expectant mothers comment that their ankles and knees feel weaker, causing them to lose their balance as the joints seem to buckle under them.

PREVENTION

You can't prevent the pregnancy-related changes in the shape of your body or the stability of your joints, but you may be able to minimize their effects with these suggestions:

What to Do

❑ Enroll in a prenatal exercise class to help strengthen your leg and ankle muscles.
❑ If you can't take a class, do foot and leg circles from a sitting position.
❑ Use the guidelines for standing and lifting described under "Backache: Prevention" on page 16.
❑ When arising from a lying, sitting, or squatting position, brace yourself by holding onto a fixed object, such as a counter top or a heavy chair.

What to Avoid

❑ Avoid activities requiring good balance, such as biking and skiing.

COMFORT

What to Do

❑ See Prevention tips on page 25.

(*See also* Dizziness, page 49; and Fainting, page 52.)

Bladder Control

One of the first signs of pregnancy is urinary frequency, or the urge to urinate often. It's also one of the most persistent complaints of expectant mothers. If you're like most women, you'll have the most trouble with this during the first and third trimesters.

One reason for urinary frequency is that during pregnancy, your body makes more urine in order to take care of your baby's waste products, as well as yours. This extra urine means your bladder fills up more often. Unfortunately, with the weight of your baby pressing against your bladder, it can't hold as much as before.

In addition to more urine and less bladder capacity, you may also experience some loss of control over the muscles that regulate the release of urine. The muscles of your pelvic floor are like a sling or hammock supporting your uterus, bladder, and other pelvic organs. As the weight of the uterus and baby increases, the hammock sags, weakening the support. Since you use these muscles when you urinate (and when you try not to urinate), this weakness makes it more difficult to control the release of urine. And, as if this weren't enough, the baby puts added pressure on your bladder, so that it can't hold as much urine as before.

PREVENTION

What to Do

❑ Practice the Kegel exercise frequently throughout the day (see page 28).
❑ Try to empty your bladder completely when you urinate. When you think you're finished urinating, place your hands on your lower abdomen and lift the baby to release any trapped urine. (Frequent urination is especially troublesome at night, when you might have to get up several times to empty your bladder. What's probably happening is this: You're lying in bed and you realize

your bladder is full. When you stand up to go to the bathroom, the baby drops down onto your bladder, trapping some urine in a portion of it. You won't be aware of that urine until you lie down again and the liquid flows toward the bottom of your bladder, where it signals you that it's time to go again.)

What to Avoid

❏ Avoid decreasing your fluid intake. This may decrease the amount of urine you have, but it will increase your risk of bladder infection and other problems.

COMFORT

What to Do

❏ Practice the Kegel frequently (see page 28) as an exercise, and use it to help control your bladder when necessary.
❏ Use a sanitary pad if leakage becomes a problem.

Episiotomy

During delivery, the pelvic floor muscles and the surrounding tissue of the *perineum* (the area between the vagina and rectum) are greatly stretched by the baby's head. Some obstetricians insist that it's necessary to make an incision in the perineum in order to prevent overstretching or tearing during the birth. Called an *episiotomy*, this incision is done for several reasons. Some doctors feel that if the tissue is allowed to overstretch, it might never regain its normal elasticity. Then, they say, in later life the woman will have difficulty because the weakened muscle will allow the bladder and uterus to drop. If the problem becomes severe, an operation called an anterior and posterior (A&P) repair may be necessary. Many childbirth educators, midwives, and physical therapists, along with some doctors and nurses, disagree. Instead, they believe that if properly exercised and strengthened before and after birth, the muscle will remain healthy and will perform

its natural function, even without an episiotomy.

Another reason for an episiotomy is that doctors say an incision is easier to suture than a tear. Numerous studies have found that episiotomies actually *increase* the risk of major perineal injury. When midwives assist women in delivering their babies, they use hot packs, oil, and massage to slowly and gently stretch and mold the perineum as the baby's head pushes against it. Midwives also encourage women to deliver in a sitting, kneeling, or side-lying postion. Those who use these techniques believe they're one reason midwives' patients often avoid tearing. Even when tearing does occur, it's usually quite superficial and simple to suture.

Whether or not you have an episiotomy, if you exercise and strengthen your perineal muscles you'll have more control over them, which will help during the birth process and will reduce your chance of bladder control problems.

EXERCISE TECHNIQUES

KEGEL

Benefits: Strengthens and tightens muscles surrounding urinary, vaginal, and rectal openings.

The figure below shows the pelvic floor muscle surrounding the outlets to the bladder, uterus, and rectum in a sort of a figure-eight formation. The Kegel helps strengthen this muscle, increasing its support and giving you more control. Here's how:

1. Tighten the muscles you use when trying to hold back urine.
2. Hold for a slow count of three.
3. Release.
4. Repeat five times.
5. Repeat the Kegel frequently throughout the day, gradually increasing the length of the count as you hold it.

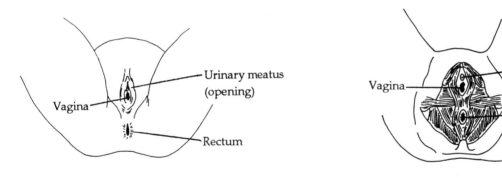

Pelvic Floor   *Muscles of the Pelvic Floor*

Comments: Try not to tighten your buttocks when doing the Kegel. The movement should be an internal one, not detected by an outside observer.

For an added benefit, practice the movement this muscle needs to make during your baby's birth. Just imagine you're on the toilet and the telephone begins to ring (and you don't have an answering machine!). You want to hurry, so you try to push the urine out forcefully. This reverse Kegel makes the muscles of the pelvic floor and lower abdomen bulge downward, and this is just the action needed to help push out your baby. Finish the reverse Kegel with a regular Kegel. (By the way, the safest place to practice the reverse Kegel is on the toilet.)

Bladder Infections

As a woman, you're far more likely to have a bladder infection, or *cystitis*, than a man is because your urinary tract is shorter and it lies close to your rectum and vagina. Now that you're pregnant, the chances of developing cystitis are even higher. Your kidneys, which filter waste products from your blood, are working harder now because your blood contains about 40 percent more fluid than before. At the same time, they're feeling pressure from the growing weight of your baby.

The two main symptoms of cystitis are *dysuria*—a burning sensation when you urinate—and urinary urgency, a recurring sense that you need to urinate immediately, even though there may not be any urine in your bladder. If you notice either or both of these symptoms, be sure to notify your doctor or midwife.

Treatment for a bladder infection usually includes antibiotics. Your doctor will choose one that is effective against the type of infection you have, and with the safest possible track record in pregnant women and their unborn children. If you're concerned about the possible effect of the medication on your baby, don't hesitate to discuss it with your doctor. But, keep in mind that the infection isn't doing you or your baby any good, and it could get worse if not treated.

Kidney Infections

If untreated, a bladder infection can spread to the kidneys, causing infection there, too. Symptoms of a kidney infection, or *pylitis*, include any or all of the following:

- ❏ Fever.
- ❏ Pain in the lower back, which worsens if you apply pressure to the area.
- ❏ Nausea and vomiting.

Notify your doctor or midwife if you suspect you may have a kidney infection. As with cystitis, antibiotics will probably be prescribed to treat the infection.

PREVENTION

What to Do

- ❏ Drink at least eight 8-ounce glasses of water daily. (Milk and real fruit juice count as water, but sodas do not. Tea counts, too, but try to limit your intake of caffeinated products.)
- ❏ Drink cranberry juice and eat citrus fruits, such as oranges, pineapples, and grapefruits. They can help change the acidity of your urine and make it difficult for bacteria to grow.
- ❏ Practice good personal hygiene. The rectum and vagina normally contain bacteria that are not found in the bladder. To avoid contaminating your bladder, clean yourself after each bowel movement or after urinating by wiping from the front to the back. And, after having intercourse, cleanse yourself by pouring warm water over your vaginal and urinary area. (Do not douche unless your doctor has told you to do so.)
- ❏ Empty your bladder completely and often.
- ❏ Empty your bladder before and after sexual intercourse to help wash away bacteria.
- ❏ Wear cotton panties, or at least a panty with a cotton crotch.

What to Avoid

- ❏ Avoid restrictive clothing, such as pantyhose or leotards, and other items that don't allow moisture to evaporate.
- ❏ Avoid feminine hygiene sprays and perfumed bubble bath or bath oil. (They can irritate delicate tissues, increasing the risk of infection.)

COMFORT

What to Do

- ❏ See Prevention tips, above.
- ❏ If urination is painful, use a squeeze bottle to spray warm water over your urinary opening *while* you urinate.
- ❏ If toilet paper irritates you, use one of the pre-moistened towelettes designed for infants.

What to Avoid

- ❏ Avoid using colored or scented toilet paper.

Bleeding

See Gum Bleeding; Nosebleeds; Vaginal Discharge.

Breast Changes

In the first weeks of pregnancy, you may experience fullness, tenderness, or tingling in your breasts, and your nipples may be so sensitive that even the gentle brushing of clothing against them feels uncomfortable. Although the tenderness usually subsides after the first trimester, your breasts continue to enlarge as they prepare for the work of producing milk after your baby is born. In order to accommodate these changes, the blood supply to your breasts increases, as you can probably see from the blue lines of your blood vessels running under the skin surface.

Some of the most noticeable changes take place in the nipples. For example, they darken during pregnancy and, although they may lighten a bit after the baby is born, they'll probably never return to their original shade. Your nipples may also protrude more now, or they may become erect more readily than before. Some pregnant women find that their nipples respond more easily to sexual intercourse and orgasm, or to the simple touch of their lover's hand. Others need only to feel cool air or the touch of clothing for erection to occur. This is your breasts' own way of preparing to nurse your baby, who will be able to grasp and suck from an erect nipple more easily than from one that is inverted. Nature does its best to see to it that every mother can properly nourish her child, so even a woman with inverted nipples may find that toward the end of pregnancy they become more erect.

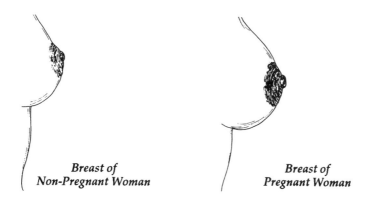

Breast of
Non-Pregnant Woman

Breast of
Pregnant Woman

One change that sometimes worries expectant mothers is something that looks like a circle of tiny nipples surrounding the *areola*, the darkened area around the nipple. Called *Montgomery's glands*, these are simply oil glands that become more prominent during pregnancy.

By the middle of pregnancy, you'll probably notice a watery secretion coming from the nipples. Called *colostrum* or *first milk*, it starts out sticky and yellow, but in late pregnancy it turns whitish and looks like watery milk. It's not unusual for colostrum to ooze, or even spurt, out when warm shower water hits your breasts or when you're sexually aroused. If you haven't noticed any colostrum, you may be able to express some by placing your index finger above the nipple and your middle finger below and using a squeeze-pull motion.

If you plan to breastfeed, colostrum will be your baby's first nourishment after he's born. Colostrum is created with your baby's health in mind. It's high in proteins and it contains important antibodies to help protect your newborn from infections. Experts also believe that colostrum helps prevent allergies in the infant.

Don't worry if you don't seem to have any colostrum. This doesn't mean you cannot produce milk. Nor does a small breast preclude a good milk supply. In fact, your baby's suckling is the most important factor in the quantity of milk you produce. The more he sucks, the more milk you'll make.

What About Nipple Preparation?

Nipple soreness is one of the most common reasons that new mothers give up on nursing; so, for years, women have been urged to do all sorts of things in order to "toughen" their nipples before the baby is born. But we know now from research and experience that these methods don't usually help and may even damage the delicate tissues of your nipples. According to Julie Stock, medical liaison for La Leche League International, correct positioning of the baby at the mother's breast is the most important factor in preventing nipple soreness and ensuring an adequate milk supply. (See page 134 for information on positioning.)

❑ If your nipples are flat or *inverted*, use a breast shell to encourage them to protrude. These are available in pharmacies and some maternity shops or from special mail-order catalogs. It's usually best to choose a shell with holes that allow moisture to evaporate.

❑ If your nipples are inverted and you feel you really must do something to prepare them, try this method, called *nipple rotation:*

Grasp the nipple between your thumb and forefinger and pull it out. You should feel only pull, no pain. Roll the nipple, in this position, between your thumb and forefinger for a couple of minutes. Afterward, soothe your nipples by expressing a few drops of colostrum and spreading it on the nipples.

(If you have inverted nipples, keep in mind that sexual breast play by your partner is a terrific way to encourage the nipples into an erection.)

COMFORT

What to Do

- ☐ Clean your breasts and nipples with plain warm water when you bathe or shower.
- ☐ Wear a well-fitting, supportive bra to reduce the pull of gravity on your breasts. (This won't prevent later sagging, but it will make you more comfortable now and may reduce the severity of stretch marks later.)
- ☐ Ease tender nipples by wearing soft-textured clothing.
- ☐ Soothe tender nipples by gently massaging with vitamin E or an unscented moisturizer. If you can easily express a few drops of colostrum, use it to soothe and protect your nipples. (Do not try to express colostrum forceably.)
- ☐ If leakage is a problem, use a cloth or disposable breast pad.

What to Avoid

- ☐ Avoid rubbing your nipples with a rough cloth or using other techniques intended to toughen nipples.
- ☐ Avoid using alcohol, soap, or perfumed creams on your nipples.

(*See also* Breast Changes, postpartal, page 130.)

Breathlessness

When I first started teaching childbirth classes, I was bothered by the sights and sounds of so many sighs and yawns from expectant mothers. Eventually, I learned that they weren't bored, they were just trying to catch a good, full breath of air.

The problem is that you're breathing for two now, so you need to inhale more oxygen and to exhale more carbon dioxide than before. At the same time, though, your growing baby is pressing your abdominal organs up toward your chest. As the pressure increases, these organs push upward against your *diaphragm,* the plate-like muscle that separates your chest cavity from your abdominal cavity. The diaphragm's function is to pull down during inhalation, making room for your lungs to expand and fill with air. When you exhale, the diaphragm relaxes up into its normal pushing postion, helping your lungs expel the air. As your baby continues to grow, your lungs won't be able to expand as fully as before because your diaphragm will have less room in which to work.

Another source of trouble involves your rib cage. Ordinarily your ribs move slightly outward when you inhale, allowing your lungs to expand in width. But in late pregnancy, your ribs are already stretched out-ward in order to make room for your diaphragm and abdominal organs, which may be nearer to your chest than your abdomen now. Although certain anatomical and physiological changes allow you to consume more oxygen, you may feel that your breathing is inhibited.

So here you are, breathing for two, but you can't get a full, complete breath of air. But you *can* do something to improve the situation.

COMFORT

What to Do

❑ Try these exercises to increase your lung capacity.
- Standing Complete Breath (page 35).
- Sitting Deep Breath (below).

What to Avoid

❑ Avoid traveling from a low altitude to a high altitude during the last half of pregnancy. (High-altitude air contains less oxygen and may increase breathing difficulty.)
❑ Avoid taking up aerobic exercise during pregnancy unless you are already accustomed to it.

EXERCISE TECHNIQUES

SITTING DEEP BREATH

Benefits: Increases lung capacity, reduces tension and fatigue, and energizes.

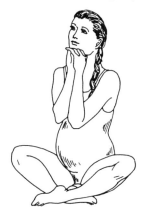

*Sitting Complete Breath —
1st Position*

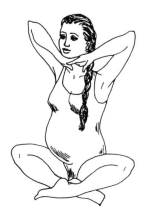

*Sitting Complete Breath —
2nd Position*

1. Sit with your legs comfortably crossed in front of you, being careful to keep one foot in front of the other. (Don't cross your ankles.)
2. Clasp your hands and place them under your chin, keeping your elbows pointed downward.
3. Inhale slowly, bringing your elbows as high as you can. Exhale slowly, extending your head back as far as possible.
4. Inhale, bringing your head forward again.
5. Exhale as you bring your elbows down to the starting position.

STANDING COMPLETE BREATH

Benefits: Increases lung capacity, helps relieve upper backache, reduces tension and fatigue, and energizes.

1. Stand with your feet comfortably apart, your hands at your sides.
2. Inhale slowly, bringing both arms up over your head until your palms touch.
3. Exhale slowly, bringing your arms back down to your sides, and letting your head drop, as though it were too heavy to hold.
4. Repeat several times, trying to inhale and exhale more slowly and prolonging the time it takes to move your arms up and down.

   Comments: If these exercises make you dizzy, sit or lie down and hold your breath for several seconds.

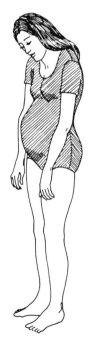
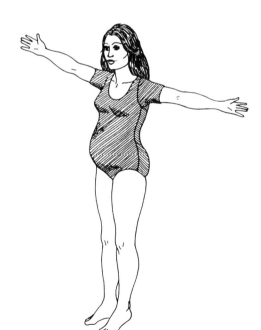
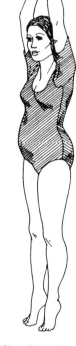

Standing Complete Breath—   *Standing Complete Breath—*   *Standing Complete Breath—*
1st Position   *2nd Position*   *3rd Position*

Constipation

If, like many expectant mothers, you've experienced recurring bouts of constipation, you know it can leave you feeling tired, bloated, and generally miserable.

Constipation during pregnancy has three main sources:

❏ Slow digestion.
❏ Pressure on the intestines.
❏ Lack of moisture.

An adult's intestinal tract consists of twenty-five feet of muscular tubing twisted and compressed into a small amount of space. When you consider how the growing uterus crowds against the intestines (see figures on pages 4 and 5), pushing them into an even smaller space, it's easy to understand why things might move along more slowly during pregnancy. And, as if that weren't enough, the hormonal changes of pregnancy slow down intestinal movement even further.

As waste moves through your body, moisture is automatically reabsorbed into the system. This means that the longer it takes the waste to move through your intestines, the harder the waste gets. And, of course, the harder it gets, the more difficult it is to expel.

PREVENTION

What to Do

❏ Take a brisk walk or swim several times a week to help stimulate your system.
❏ Exercise regularly, making sure to include these exercises that allow your abdominal muscles to massage your intestinal tract:
  • Pelvic Tilt (page 10).
  • Forward Bend (page 20).
  • Buttocks Curl (page 11).

❏ Drink warm liquids to stimulate intestinal activity. It's especially helpful to start the day with a warm drink. If you're not nauseated in the morning, squeeze the juice of half a lemon into a cup of hot water and sweeten it with a little honey.
❏ Drink *at least* eight 8-ounce glasses of water daily. This includes other liquids, such as milk or juice. Tea counts, too, but try to limit

your intake of this and other caffeine products. (Sodas don't count as liquids—they may actually increase your need for fluid.) To find out how much liquid you're drinking each day, pour eight glasses of water into a covered pitcher in the morning. Throughout the day, take your water from this container. If you drink another liquid, pour an equal amount of water out of the pitcher. At the end of the day, measure any remaining water to see how much you actually drank.

❑ Add bulk to your diet by eating plenty of whole grains and raw, unpeeled fruits and vegetables. (If you don't like raw vegetables, try lightly steaming them.)

COMFORT

What to Do

❑ See Prevention tips, above.
❑ Keep a small footstool in the bathroom. When you're on the toilet, rest your feet on the footstool to provide better leverage and prevent unnecessary straining.

What to Avoid

❑ Avoid commercial laxatives, unless prescribed by your birth attendant. If prescribed, take only as a temporary measure. Do not continue taking laxatives on a regular basis—doing so will make your intestines dependent on them.
❑ Avoid enemas, unless prescribed by your birth attendant. If prescribed, use only as a temporary, one-time remedy.

(*See also* Gas, page 61.)

Contractions

"During the last trimester, my abdomen would bulge and harden on one side or in the middle. At first, it lasted only ten or twenty seconds; but later, it sometimes lasted longer. I thought it was the baby butting me with his head; but, when I attended Lamaze classes, I was surprised to find out that these were really contractions."

Towards the middle or end of pregnancy, you may be surprised to notice your uterus harden for a moment, and then soften again. What you're feeling is a portion of your uterus contracting as it prepares for the work of labor. Called *Braxton-Hicks*, these practice contractions may be brought on by seemingly unrelated activities, such as housework or vigorous exercise. Braxton-Hicks contractions may also occur during or after intercourse, especially if you experience orgasm. There's usually no need for alarm, though—in a healthy woman having a normal pregnancy, these Braxton-Hicks contractions will not become real contractions until the time is right.

If you're a first-time mother, or *primip*, you may not notice Braxton-Hicks contractions until the last month. In fact, you may not be aware of them at all unless someone mentions them. If this is your second or third baby, you'll probably feel them much earlier than you did the first time because you know what they feel like. You'll probably feel more of these contractions, too, because the experienced uterus tends to practice more, accomplishing more work ahead of time than before. Toward the end of pregnancy, these practice contractions are often referred to as *false labor*, but they actually can help the cervix start to dilate and shorten, or efface, so that the baby can be born.

Braxton-Hicks contractions are *supposed* to be painless. At least that's what the textbooks say. But some expectant mothers have told me their Braxton-Hicks contractions are quite uncomfortable, especially when they continue for an hour or longer. You can ease the discomfort of these practice contractions with the same techniques used for labor. In fact, it's a great way to practice what you're learning in childbirth preparation classes.

COMFORT

What to Do

❑ Use these massage techniques to reduce discomfort:

- Simple Effleurage (page 40).
- Valentine Effleurage (page 41).
- Partner's Effleurage (page 42).

❑ Use The Balloon relaxation technique. (See page 163.)

❑ Take advantage of Braxton-Hicks contractions to practice the breathing and relaxation techniques you're learning in your childbirth class.

❑ If you think you might be in labor, rest to conserve your energy and refer to the inset on page 39 ("Am I in Labor Yet?").

Am I in Labor Yet?

False labor can occur on and off for days or even weeks; but, as time passes, you'll notice the contractions increasing in frequency and becoming longer, stronger, and more regular. Most women notice several of these symptoms within a week of the onset of true labor:

❑ Sudden weight loss of two or three pounds.
❑ Burst of energy.
❑ Increased vaginal discharge.
❑ Increased Braxton-Hicks contractions.
❑ Sensation of pressure or heaviness in the pelvis or lower back.
❑ Nausea/vomiting.
❑ Diarrhea.

To determine whether you're in labor, compare your contractions with the characteristics mentioned below:

False Labor

❑ Contractions usually harden only a portion of the uterus.
❑ Contractions usually lack pattern, regularity, or symmetry.
❑ Change of activity usually stops contractions.
❑ Contractions may get longer, stronger, and closer together, but one or more of these features is usually missing.

True Labor

❑ Contractions usually harden entire uterus.
❑ Contractions usually follow a pattern and become regular and symmetrical.
❑ Change of activity will not stop true labor, although tension may slow it; walking may increase the strength of contractions.

❑ Contractions usually get longer, stronger, and closer together.

Call your birth attendant or go to the hospital when the contractions have been coming every five minutes for an hour if this is your first baby, or every ten minutes for an hour if this is not your first. (Time contractions from the beginning of one to the beginning of the next one.) If you think the bag of waters has broken, call your birth attendant or go to the hospital; do not wait for contractions.

Of course, we all know someone who arrived at the hospital, ready to have the baby, only to discover that her contractions stopped as soon as she was admitted. If this happens to you, it may simply mean that the excitement and anxiety of being admitted to the hospital have created enough tension to cause a temporary lull in the birth process. Once you've settled into your room and have begun to relax, the contractions will probably resume.

On the other hand, you may have experienced a false start. Even though the contractions got longer and stronger and more frequent, they weren't ready to continue. False starts are more common among women who've already had a baby because they tend to experience more false labor, making it harder to tell whether or not they're really in labor. These moms may also be more eager to get to the hospital because they know a second or third labor is likely to be shorter than a first.

Most women feel embarrassed about being sent home after thinking they were in labor. They worry that they've behaved foolishly and that they've bothered the nurses and birth attendant. But, even the experts can't tell for certain whether you're in labor until they've examined you. And they still may have to wait to see if the contractions and dilatation continue before determining that you definitely are in labor.

What to Avoid

❏ If you think labor may be starting—avoid eating a heavy or spicy meal; avoid physical exertion in order to conserve energy; avoid taking any medication without consulting your birth attendant.

LABOR TIPS

Painful Contractions:

Most women find that while effleurage helps reduce discomfort in false or early labor, it takes more pressure to deal with the discomfort of active labor. You can still use the patterns described on pages 40-42, but you'll need to press more firmly. As you do, the controlled breathing and rhythmic movement of your hands, combined with the warmth and pressure they provide, will help to ease the discomfort of contractions.

Long Labor/Plateau

Use The Balloon relaxation technique (page 163) to relieve pain and tension when labor is long and the contractions are rough or if you hit a *plateau,* a period during labor when the contractions keep coming, but there's no progress toward dilating the cervix or moving the baby down toward the birth canal. A plateau is most likely to occur when your cervix is dilated between three and seven centimeters. In addition to using The Balloon, here are several other remedies that can help you overcome a plateau:

❏ Change your position every half hour or so.
❏ If you can walk comfortably, do so.
❏ Remember to empty your bladder every hour or so, to give your baby room to move down.
❏ You or your partner may want to try a technique called "nipple stimulation." When you gently stroke your nipples, your pituitary gland releases oxytocin, a hormone that stimulates your uterus to contract.

MASSAGE TECHNIQUES

ABDOMINAL EFFLEURAGE

Effleurage is a French word for a light massage done with the fingertips. You can do effleurage through clothing, but it feels better on bare skin with an application of talc or lotion to reduce friction. For best relaxation, inhale as your hands move up your abdomen and exhale as they move down.

Benefits: A light touch relaxes during false or early labor. (For pain relief and relaxation during active or late labor, switch to firm pressure.)

1. Sit in a comfortable position, resting your elbows on the arms of a chair or on a pillow. Lift and then drop your shoulders to let them relax.
2. Place both hands just above your pubic bone and start rubbing your tummy, using a slow, gentle wrist motion to move your fingers up and down your abdomen.

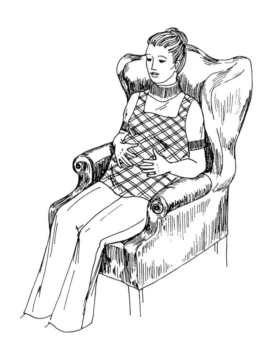

Abdominal Effleurage

VALENTINE EFFLEURAGE

Benefits: A light touch relaxes during false or early labor. (For pain relief and relaxation during active or late labor, switch to firm pressure.)

1. Start in a comfortable, well-supported position.
2. Place the fingers of both hands just above the pubic bone and then draw them outward and upward, as though tracing a large heart on your tummy.
3. When you reach the top of your abdomen, bring both hands to the center and then slide them down the middle in a straight line, all the way to the starting point.
4. Continue repeating the pattern as long as desired.

PARTNER'S EFFLEURAGE

(These directions are written for your partner.)

Benefits: A light touch relaxes during false or early labor. (For pain relief and relaxation during active or late labor, switch to firm pressure.)

To effleurage the abdomen while the woman is sitting on the bed or floor:

1. Sit behind her, with your legs outstretched so that she can lean back and relax on your chest.
2. Reach around her and massage her abdomen by moving your hands up and down or in a heart-shaped pattern, as described for Abdominal Effleurage or Valentine Effleurage (see pages 40 and 41).

To effleurage her abdomen while she is lying on her side:

1. Sit or stand behind her.
2. Place one hand on the far side of her abdomen at a point near the bed.
3. Slowly pull your hand up toward yourself, applying firm, gentle pressure.
4. Just before the first hand reaches the near side of her abdomen, place your other hand on the far side and begin moving it upward. (One hand should always be touching her abdomen.)
5. Continue stroking her abdomen this way, so that one hand ends a stroke just as the other hand begins. Keep the motion slow and rhythmic.

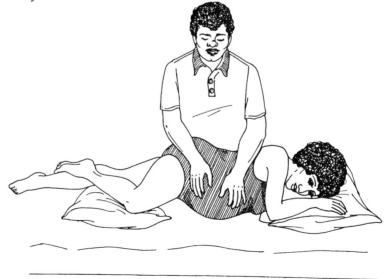

Partner's Effleurage

Cramps, Abdominal or Uterine

See Contractions; Groin Pain.

Cramps, Leg

Leg cramps, or charley horses, are a common complaint during the last half of pregnancy. This sudden stabbing pain that grabs your calf usually strikes at night when you're sleeping, or in the morning as you stretch your legs and get ready to stand up. If you're like me, your first reaction is probably to rub your leg, or to yell for your husband to wake up and rub it for you.

No one knows what causes leg cramps, but some experts believe it's related to an imbalance between the two minerals calcium and phosphorus.

PREVENTION

What to Do

❏ Do these exercises daily, preferably before going to bed:

- Leg Stretch (page 45).
- Wall Push-Ups (page 46).

❏ Include 1,200 milligrams of calcium in your daily diet. You can get this from four average servings of milk products. If you're unable to drink milk, try a calcium supplement.

❏ When possible, avoid the food additive *phosphate*, which is found in carbonated beverages and in many processed foods.

❏ If you are drinking more milk than is required, and decreasing the phosphates has not helped, try decreasing your milk intake to the required four servings.

What to Avoid

❏ Avoid pointing your toes. This movement contracts the very muscles that cause leg cramps.

❑ Avoid taking too much calcium. Both too much and too little calcium can cause cramps.

COMFORT

What to Do

❑ Apply heat to help relieve a leg cramp or to reduce any soreness left afterwards. Try a heating pad or a nice, long soak in warm water.

❑ Relieve the spasm by flexing your foot, which will stretch the muscles in the opposite direction and help them relax. Simply standing up accomplishes this, but if you prefer a gentler, less abrupt method, try this:

1. Sit up in bed with your leg outstretched and use one hand to gently push down on your knee.
2. With the other hand, grasp the sole of your foot and gently pull it toward you.

What to Avoid

❑ Avoid taking aspirin or ibuprofen.

LABOR TIPS

Muscle cramps, especially in the legs, are sometimes a problem during labor. When this happens, it's often due to improper breathing, or *hyperventilation*. This can happen if you breathe too rapidly and deeply. When you hyperventilate, you don't get a good exchange of oxygen and carbon dioxide in your lungs and blood, and neither does your baby. As a result, you may feel dizzy and light-headed and you may experience muscle cramps or feel numbness or tingling in your hands or feet.

Hyperventilation often leads to a feeling of panic and a fear of not getting enough air. Follow these steps to relieve it:

1. Take a deep breath and hold it in for as long as you can.
2. Let the air out very slowly, through pursed lips or with a hiss.
3. Ask your partner to give you the Soothing Touch massage (page 69).
4. Try to breathe at a relaxed pace of about eight to twelve breaths per minute.
5. Use The Swing (page 82) or The Balloon (page 163) to help you relax and focus.

To prevent hyperventilation and other problems, do not breathe faster than twice your normal rate or slower than half your normal rate.

EXERCISE TECHNIQUES

LEG STRETCH

Benefits: Helps prevent or relieve leg cramps and improves flexibility.

1. Sit on the floor and stretch your right leg out to the side while folding your left leg in.
2. Face forward and bend at the waist to the right side so that your upper body is over your right leg.
3. Use your right hand to grasp your right foot (see the figure below). If you can't do this comfortably, reach for your ankle or for a point slightly closer to your body.
4. Hold this position for ten seconds, trying to keep your right knee as close to the floor as possible.
5. Relax and release the stretch.
6. Repeat on the other side.

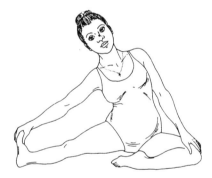

Leg Stretch

Comments: You may feel uncomfortable, especially at the back of your leg, when you first do this stretch. If it actually hurts, you may have reached too far. But be sure you know the difference between pain and stretch. If you're not used to giving your muscles a good, healthy stretch, this may be an unfamiliar feeling at first, but it isn't necessarily a painful one. You can be more comfortable and stretch farther if after assuming the stretch position, you consciously think about what parts of your body are tense. These tight muscles are holding you back and making you uncomfortable, so let go of them. As you hold the stretch, take a mental trip through your body, moving from head to toe and letting go of each part as you think of it. Once everything is as relaxed as possible, try to stretch a little farther before finishing the exercise. Afterwards, it feels good to shake your legs vigorously.

WALL PUSH-UPS

Benefits: Helps prevent or relieve leg cramps and strengthens arm and chest muscles.

1. Stand facing the wall, with your feet about eighteen to twenty-four inches away from it.
2. Place your hands on the wall for support, with your fingers pointing either upward or toward the center.
3. Inhale and bend your elbows, leaning your body toward the wall. (Keep your legs straight and your heels on the floor.)
4. Exhale while pushing yourself away from the wall, back to the starting position.
5. Repeat several times, always inhaling as you move toward the wall and exhaling as you push away from it.

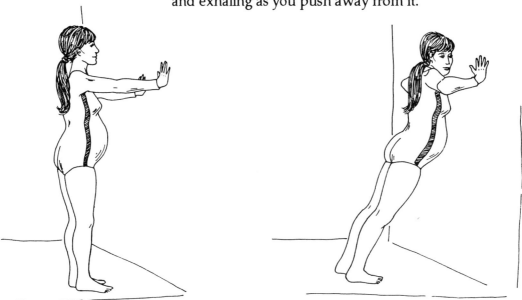

Wall Push-Ups—1st Position   *Wall Push-Ups—2nd Position*

Comments: If you have a hard time keeping your heels on the floor during this exercise, move your feet a little closer to the wall. As you practice, your calf muscles will begin to stretch more easily, allowing you to stand farther away. After a while, this exercise may not provide enough of a challenge for you. To increase both the challenge and the benefits, move your starting position a few inches back from the wall. For good support, you'll need to adjust the placement of your hands so that the farther away from the wall you stand, the farther apart your hands are. As you move farther from the wall, you may also find it more comfortable to place your hands so that the fingers face inward.

Cravings

"My wife craved watermelon in the dead of winter, and I almost went nuts trying to find some. I brought her apples and oranges, and I even came up with some kiwi fruit, but no watermelon. Next time, we're planning a summer pregnancy!"

Husbands kid about them, mothers-in-law tell you to yield to them, and doctors tell you they're all in your head. Cravings can hit a pregnant woman at any time. You may find that you crave a particular food all through pregnancy, or you may never have a single craving the entire time.

What causes cravings? Some experts think they're your body's way of supplying nutrients missing from your diet. For example, if you crave lots of oranges or grapefruits, it may be your body's way of saying you need more vitamin C. On the other hand, you may just need a higher concentration of flavor because during pregnancy your taste threshold increases. Delicately seasoned foods may seem bland now, while tart citrus fruits may taste just right. Other experts say a woman who craves food is really craving more attention. In other words, if you express a strong desire for exotic food or out-of-season fruit, you're really asking your husband if he loves you enough to bring you what you want.

What about the woman who wakes up hungry for pizza or egg rolls in the middle of the night? Late-night hunger pangs hit everybody at one time or another, but they happen more often during pregnancy. It takes extra calories to fill your needs and those of your baby, and midnight hunger attacks are probably your natural response to this increased demand.

Some cravings have a cultural origin. This is especially true of *pica*, a desire to eat a nonfood substance. The word "pica" comes from the Latin for "magpie," a bird that is said to have an eclectic appetite. An expectant mother who was working on her master's degree once asked me, "When can I stop eating the dirt?" She explained that her mother had been sending her sterile dirt from Georgia since the beginning of her pregnancy. Her mother hadn't said why she should eat it, and the woman didn't crave it or even like its taste. But all the women in her family ate dirt when they were pregnant, so she did, too. And, while other members of her childbirth class were amazed that she'd willingly eaten dirt, she was amazed that they hadn't.

The most common nonfood items a pregnant woman might crave are dirt, clay, chalk, ashes, cornstarch, and dry laundry starch. While it may be difficult to believe that anyone would eat these things, certain ethnic groups accept it as a common practice in the belief that it will help ensure the baby's health or an easier birth. Of course, this isn't true. In fact, some of these items may contain pollutants or contaminants that could harm you and your baby. To make things worse, they don't provide any vitamins, protein, or other life-sustaining properties and, if eaten in large quantities, they can interfere with your health by decreasing your appetite for the good food you and your baby need.

As mentioned in the section on "Anemia," a persistent craving for ice is more common in women who are anemic, so be sure to let your doctor or midwife know if you find yourself eating a lot of ice. If you have a persistent craving for another nonfood substance, talk with your midwife, or ask your physician to refer you to a dietitian who can discuss your diet with you and help you deal with the craving.

PREVENTION

What to Do

❑ Eat a well-balanced diet that includes plenty of fruits and vegetables, whole grains, fish, chicken, meats, cheese, and milk products. (This may prevent cravings in some cases.)

❑ To prevent late-night cravings, try a light snack and a glass of milk before going to bed.

Fact or Fiction?

If you don't give in and satisfy a craving, your baby will be "marked." This myth is usually told with the story of a distant relative who didn't heed a craving for strawberries and ended up giving birth to a baby with a red, strawberry-shaped birthmark. Although there's no truth to this belief, it's so old and so widely held that it has become part of the language in at least two countries. The French word *envie* and the Italian word *voglia* both can be used to mean either a craving or a birthmark.

Cravings are your baby's way of telling you what food he wants. Not really. What you eat enters your baby's system through the bloodstream, so he doesn't care what it tastes like. And since the food has been reduced to its basic nutrients by the time it reaches your baby, he can't distinguish one food from another.

If you crave red meat, it means your baby is a boy. This is an old myth, but it keeps cropping up, especially when older relatives come to visit. The reverse of this myth is that you can increase your chances of having a boy if you eat lots of red meat. But since your baby's sex was determined at the time of conception, this is right only 50 percent of the time.

COMFORT

What to Do

❏ Indulge yourself occasionally. If you're hungry for pizza with the works, followed by a hot fudge sundae, it's okay to indulge yourself once every week or two. But if you crave these high-fat, high-sodium foods more often, try to satisfy your hunger with a meatless pizza, along with ice milk or low-fat frozen yogurt.

What to Avoid

❏ Avoid eating nonfood substances.
❏ Avoid filling up on one type of food. You and your baby need the variety of a balanced diet.
❏ Avoid restricting your caloric intake. You need to gain at least twenty-five to thirty-five pounds to give your baby the optimum chance of being big and healthy. It's okay to splurge now and then, as long as you eat right the rest of the time.

(*See also* Weight Gain, page 115.)

Cystitis

See Bladder Infections.

Dizziness

Occasional dizziness is fairly common during pregnancy, especially if you sit up or stand up too fast. You're more likely to experience dizziness in late pregnancy, when extra fluid in your bloodstream makes blood flow more slowly. As a result, your vascular system may take longer to adjust to a position change. If you stand up too fast, the blood that was circulating through your brain may flow down from it faster than replacement blood can flow back up to it. This lack of sufficient blood in your brain leaves you momentarily dizzy, but it usually passes quickly and is rarely cause for alarm. If the dizziness persists, though, tell your doctor or midwife.

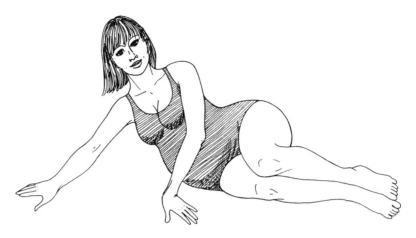

Arising From a Lying Position

PREVENTION

What to Do

❑ Move slowly when changing positions so that your blood can catch up with you.

COMFORT

What to Do

❑ Lie quietly on your left side. This will improve your circulation almost immediately, and you should feel better in a matter of minutes.

❑ If you can't lie down, try to sit with your head lowered.

(*See also* Balance Disturbances, page 25; and Fainting, page 52.)

Dreams

"I have this recurring dream where my wife drives away in our brand new car. As she's leaving, she waves at me and calls out, 'Don't worry. I'll send you the baby.'"

This expectant father's dream scared him because he thought it might be an omen that his wife would actually leave him. But after discussing it with her, he realized the dream was only an expression of his concern for her. The doctor had said she would probably need a cesarean delivery and that her husband wouldn't be allowed in the room with her. This left him feeling helpless and afraid that she might die and leave him alone with the baby.

Disturbing dreams are common among expectant mothers and fathers. It's only natural for the thoughts and fears that concern you by day to manifest themselves in your dreams by night. For example, you might dream that your baby isn't healthy, or that your labor is long and difficult. Or, as with the father quoted above, some of your dreams may not contain clear messages and they may confuse you.

Of course, not every dream is a revelation of your innermost thoughts. Some elements of dreams are simply left over from what you saw, heard, or did the day before. But a recurring dream is usually a message from your brain that you need to sort out something.

COMFORT

What to Do

❑ Talk over recurring or disturbing dreams with your partner. If you don't feel comfortable doing this, talk to your childbirth educator.

What to Avoid

❑ Avoid putting too much meaning or importance on your dreams. Keep in mind that dreams in which there's something wrong with the baby are very common among expectant mothers. But these dreams don't have any special significance. Of course, some babies *are* born with problems. But, so far, I've never had a new mother tell me that her dreams about birth defects or other complications had actually come true.

(*See also* Insomnia, page 79; Mood Changes, page 83; and Sexual Adjustments, page 98.)

Edema

See Swelling.

Fainting

On television it's easy to tell when a woman is pregnant—she faints. Of course, if you're watching a soap opera, fainting might also foreshadow a mysterious and fatal illness. (Or, if the show needs the ratings, it might mean she's both pregnant and about to develop a mysterious and fatal illness.)

In real life, though, it's unusual for a woman to faint just because she's pregnant. Before actually fainting, you'd probably feel light-headed and dizzy and your field of vision might seem to narrow, as though you were looking at things through a tunnel. Like dizziness, fainting is related to the circulatory changes pregnancy brings. As the volume of fluid in your bloodstream increases, the rate of flow slows down, making it harder for your system to adjust to a rapid change in position. If you stand up or sit up too quickly, the blood rushes away from your brain faster than replacement blood flows back up to it.

If you do faint, anyone who is with you can help by staying there and keeping you warm. It's usually best if they don't try to move you. After all, fainting usually leaves you in a prone position, which is exactly what was needed to restore proper blood flow to your brain.

Be sure to let your doctor or midwife know if you experience a fainting spell. If you actually fall down, you should notify her right away and ask whether she wants to examine you and your baby. With all that amniotic fluid, your child is pretty well protected, but it never hurts to check it out.

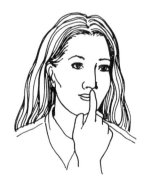

*Pressure Point to
Relieve Fainting*

PREVENTION

What to Do

❑ Take your time when changing from a lying position to a sitting one or from sitting to standing.

❑ If you feel a fainting spell beginning, you may be able to stop it by using your thumbnail or fingernail to apply sixty seconds of pressure to the skin just above the center of the upper lip.

What to Avoid

❑ Avoid prolonged standing.

❑ Avoid sitting in one position for a long time.

COMFORT

What to Do

To relieve fainting:

- ❑ Lie down on your left side for a while. (This improves circulation by taking the weight of the uterus off the vena cava, a large blood vessel that brings blood from the legs back up to the heart.)
- ❑ If no couch or bed is available, and if you're able, place your head down between your knees for a few moments until the feeling passes.
- ❑ Apply thumbnail pressure to the skin just above the center of your upper lip.
- ❑ Place a cold wet cloth on your forehead or on the back of your neck.

What to Avoid

- ❑ Never throw water into the face of a person who has fainted.
- ❑ Avoid immediately resuming physical activity.

(*See also* Dizziness, page 49.)

Fatigue

"The worst thing about being pregnant is that I'm tired all the time."

"My wife and I used to play tennis several times a week and go dancing every Saturday night. Now all she does is sleep."

Most women experience a great deal of fatigue during the first trimester of pregnancy. It's your body's way of telling you to slow down and take it easy during these crucial months of your baby's development. If this is your first pregnancy, you should get most of your energy back during the second trimester. But later, as your baby gets heavier and you move into the final weeks of pregnancy, you'll probably slow down again. Remember, being pregnant means carrying an extra twenty-five or thirty pounds everywhere you go. If your partner or your friends complain about your being so tired, take them to the store and challenge them to carry a twenty-five-pound sack of dog food or garden soil around for a few minutes. Then remind them that you do it twenty-four hours a day.

Other causes of fatigue during pregnancy include anemia, slower blood flow, and shortness of breath.

COMFORT

Fatigue is a natural and normal aspect of pregnancy. It can't be prevented, but the suggestions below can help reduce it.

What to Do

❑ Choose one of the following activities and do it for twenty to thirty minutes three or four times a week:

- Walking.
- Swimming.
- Bicycling. (Use a stationary bike if you're past the sixth month or if you feel unsure about your sense of balance.)

❑ Enroll in a prenatal exercise class.

❑ During your workday, take several short breaks to stretch and to do foot circles and Arm Reaches (page 59).

❑ Be sure your diet includes a generous supply of *proteins*, such as fish, cheese, poultry, and legumes, and *carbohydrates*, such as whole grains, fruits, and raw or lightly-steamed vegetables.

❑ Keep a ready supply of nutritious snacks such as these on hand:

- High-fiber, low-salt crackers.
- Fruits and juices.
- Crudites (raw vegetables cut into snack-size pieces).
- Cheese, milk, and yogurt.
- Cold chicken or turkey.
- Peanuts.

❑ Take an iron supplement daily and include iron-rich foods in your diet. (See pages 14 and 15 for food sources of iron.)

❑ Lie with your feet elevated above the level of your heart for at least fifteen minutes. Do this several times a day to improve blood flow throughout your body. (If lying on your back makes you dizzy or light-headed, turn to your left side.)

❑ Add an afternoon nap to your schedule.

❑ Be patient with yourself and listen when your body tells you it's time to rest.

❑ Buy a rocking chair and use it. The gentle and continuous motion of your legs as you rock will improve circulation. It's also great for relieving tension and backache.

What to Avoid

❏ Avoid medications advertised for increasing energy or for reducing sleepiness.
❏ Avoid excessive caffeine intake.

LABOR TIPS

Labor is exactly what its name implies: hard work. And in labor, as in anything that requires long hours of physical and mental effort, fatigue is often a major problem. Fatigue decreases your ability to concentrate and relax and magnifies every pain or discomfort you feel. Here's how to fight labor fatigue:

❏ Get as much rest as possible during the last weeks of pregnancy. Don't give in to those last-minute urges to clean out your desk or rearrange the nursery.
❏ During early labor, drink an herbal tea, such as peppermint, spearmint, or lemon, sweetened with honey or sugar.
❏ Suck on ice chips.
❏ Ask your partner to give you one of the back massages described in the section on "Backache." (A good back rub can be quite an energizer. As one of the moms in my class told me, "During labor I was exhausted and I told my husband I couldn't go on. But then he started doing pressure point massage up and down my spine and I could actually feel his energy flowing through his hands into my body.")

(*See also* Anemia, page 13.)

Fetal Activity

Years from now, when you look back on this pregnancy, there are several events that will probably be highlighted in your memories: the day you first learned you were pregnant; the first time you heard your baby's heartbeat; and, perhaps the most memorable of all—the first time you felt your baby move.

If this is your first baby, you'll probably become aware of your baby's movements during the fourth month of pregnancy. On the other hand, if you've already had a baby, you'll probably feel fetal activity in the third month because you know how it feels. This first noticeable move-ment is called *quickening,* which is an old term that refers to someone being brought back to life. This word was used because in ancient times, fetal activity was the only real indicator that the baby was alive. Today we know that your baby starts moving long before then—prob-ably by the eighth week of pregnancy. Although his movements become stronger as he grows, it's easy to mistake these early flutterings   for gas or intestinal activity. (When I was expecting my first child, I remember thinking that it felt as though bubbles or butterflies were brushing against me from inside. It was several days before I realized my baby was the one doing the brush-ing.)

Expectant parents respond to fetal activity in a variety of ways. Some say it reassures them, while others find it disturbing. But, no matter   how you feel about all the activity going on inside you, it definitely brings home the fact that there really is a baby, and you really are becoming a mother.

KEEPING A RECORD OF YOUR BABY'S ACTIVITY

If you want to keep a record of your baby's activity, set aside a twelve-hour period, beginning at the same time each day. Choose a time when you won't be focusing heavily on work and, of course, when you won't be sleeping. Then, while going about your regular routine, make it a point to notice your baby's movements. As soon as you feel one, write down the time.

Keep doing this until you have recorded ten movements, and then stop. It may take only an hour or two to accumulate ten movements, or it may take the full twelve hours. Call your doctor or midwife if you cannot detect at least ten movements in twelve hours. (While this is the generally ac-cepted guideline, your birth attendant may recommend a different kick-rate or time limit.)

IF DADDY DOESN'T FEEL THE BABY KICK

"I just started feeling the baby move last week, but every time I ask Dave to come feel it, the kicking stops. Now he's convinced the baby doesn't like him."

Even though you can feel the baby move by the fourth month, it may be another month before your husband can. After all, he's trying to feel the baby through your abdomen and uterus and all that amniotic fluid. What usually happens is that you call your husband to come quickly and feel the baby every time you notice a kick or jab. Of course, by the time he places his hand on your abdomen, the activity usually has stopped. It's only natural for a father to feel frustrated, and some have asked me if the baby's behavior is a sign of rejection. The answer, of course, is "No"—the baby probably just needed to stretch a little, and by the time the father got there, he had settled down. Or maybe the warmth and pressure of his hand on your abdomen relaxed the baby and put him to sleep.

All these are sensible explanations of why dad has trouble feeling the baby move, but my favorite theory comes from an expectant father who said, "I think my baby really likes me. He's already playing hide-and-seek with me!"

About Fetal Activity

TYPES OF FETAL ACTIVITY

Rolling. This is what you feel when your baby is trying to turn around. These movements will become less frequent as your baby grows bigger and runs out of space to maneuver.

Sharp and short. Otherwise known as a "swift kick," this happens when your baby kicks with his knees or feet, or when he stretches out his elbows or hands. Quick movements may also be caused by your baby's "rooting reflex" as he turns his head from side to side in search of his thumb. (Yes, some babies are natural-born thumbsuckers!)

Hiccups. These feel just as you would imagine–short, jumping sensations in your abdomen that occur at fairly regular intervals. In an unborn child, they probably come from drinking too much amniotic fluid. As a result, the baby's full stomach presses on his diaphragm, which reacts with the spasms we know as hiccups. Unfortunately, none of the usual remedies work. You'll just have to wait until your baby digests the excess fluid in his stomach.

Tingling. In late pregnancy, you may notice a tingling sensation in the upper part of the vagina, near the cervix. Some experts think this is caused by early changes in the cervix as it prepares for labor. Others believe the tingling comes from your baby's efforts to prepare for his big day. During the birth your baby will have to duck his head under your pubic bone and then lift it again to make his exit. In the last weeks of pregnancy, he practices this maneuver by pushing his head against your cervix. This places pressure on the nerves in the area, and may be what causes the tingling sensation.

Stretching and pushing. As your baby grows and begins to run out of space, you may feel him stretching out to give his muscles a break, or pushing against the uterine wall, as if he's trying to make more room.

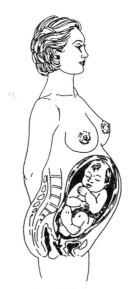

Breech Baby

Breathing. Although you probably can't feel it, your baby's chest moves in and out as though he were breathing. Since he's getting all his oxygen from you now, he's not really breathing; he's just exercising the necessary muscles so they'll be ready when it's time for him to breathe on his own.

Foot-in-the-ribs syndrome. This isn't really a fetal activity. In fact, it seems to be the result of fetal *inactivity.* It happens in late pregnancy when your baby finds a comfortable position that leaves you feeling like his foot is wedged between two of your ribs.

WHAT DOES FETAL ACTIVITY TELL YOU ABOUT YOUR BABY?

During late pregnancy the location of activity gives you clues about your baby's position. For example, if you notice most of the kicking on one side, he's probably facing that side. But, if you feel most of the kicking in the front, he's probably facing forward, with his back against your spine.

If your baby is lying with his head down toward the cervix, you'll notice the strongest kicking in the upper part of your abdomen, where his feet are. But if he's in a breech position, with his buttocks or feet near the cervix, you may feel his kicking against your bladder and rectum. (Or as one mother said, "It feels like the baby is tap-dancing on my bladder!") And when your breech baby stretches out to get more comfortable, it probably will feel like someone is pushing a cantaloupe up under your stomach and diaphragm.

You can also learn about your baby's responses to certain situations by paying attention to what makes him move and how. Some moms report increased fetal activity every time they practice relaxation-breathing. Childbirth educators often attribute this to an increased flow of oxygen to the baby, making him feel extra peppy. (On the other hand, some babies get as relaxed as their moms and fall asleep during practice sessions.)

Some babies are more susceptible to outside stimuli than others, and one baby's reactions will differ from that of another. For example, some will react to loud voices by moving, while others will become very still. You may also notice that your baby is more active when certain types of music are played. One expectant mother told me that her very active baby settled down whenever she attended the club where her husband's rock band played. On the other hand, I had to advise one mother to take a temporary leave from her job in a country-western band because her unborn baby reacted violently to the noise. (Throughout the last three months of my pregnancy, my son kicked me in perfect rhythm to the hymns we sang in church. He's turned out to have a great ear for music and has taught himself to play several difficult pieces by Beethoven.)

Your baby's activity is an important indicator of how healthy he is, especially in the last months of pregnancy. When quickening first occurs, you may notice only a few movements a day. The number increases as your baby grows and as you become aware of the different ways in which he moves. Each baby's pattern is different—some seem to move about all the time, while others are content with an occasional kick or stretch. But once your baby has established a routine, you should notice at least ten movements every twelve hours. Fewer could mean you and your baby are undernourished or tired, or it could mean he has a problem.

Even though your baby's activity can warn of problems, you shouldn't be preoccupied with it. Keep in mind that fetal movement is more than just a warning system; it's a form of communication through which your baby learns about you and tells you about himself. It's also an important part of the bonding process. So the next time he kicks you in the rib or dances on your bladder, remember, he's just trying to get to know you better.

COMFORT

What to Do

❑ Do Arm Reaches (page 59) if your baby is lying in a position that puts pressure on your diaphragm and makes it difficult to breathe, or if he seems to have his foot stuck in your ribs. (If this is your first baby, this type of discomfort should go away in the last weeks of pregnancy, when your baby settles down into your pelvis in preparation for birth. If this is not your first baby, he may not drop into the pelvis until labor has started.)

❏ If too much fetal activity keeps you awake at night, try changing positions. If this doesn't help, try Abdominal Effleurage (see page 40). (A number of fathers have proudly told me how they help their baby settle down and sleep at night by gently massaging the mother's abdomen.)

EXERCISE TECHNIQUES

ARM REACHES

Benefits: Eases shortness of breath and indigestion, may encourage baby to move to a position that is more comfortable for you, reduces tension and fatigue, and energizes.

1. Inhale deeply while slowly stretching one arm high over your head.
2. Exhale deeply while slowly bringing the arm back down.
3. Repeat several times with each arm.

Finger Numbness

During late pregnancy, some women experience occasional numbness and tingling in their fingers. This condition, which is sometimes accompanied by stiffness in the finger joints, is called *carpal tunnel syndrome* because it's caused by pressure on the carpal nerve in your wrist. The pressure comes from the normal, pregnancy-related changes in the fluid and blood flow in the tissues of your arms. This problem most often occurs in the morning, after your arms have been inactive for hours. You'll notice it especially if you sleep on your arm. If you find it bothersome, try the comfort measures on this page, which are designed to relieve the discomfort by reducing the swelling in your hands. *If your hands are noticeably swollen, and if these measures don't relieve it, notify your physician or midwife.*

PREVENTION

What to Avoid

❏ Avoid sleeping on your arm. (See figure on page 80 for how to sleep on your side without lying on your arm.)

FACT OR FICTION?

"My first two babies were boys, and when I was pregnant they kicked me all day long. This one is much quieter and gentler, so I just know she's a girl."

One of the most popular myths of pregnancy is that you can determine the baby's sex by the amount of fetal activity. While expecting my daughter, Amy, I attended a party where one woman said, "Oh, you're carrying low. That means it's a boy." Two minutes later I was approached by another woman who enthusiastically informed me, "You're carrying low. That means you're going to have a girl!" These forecasts that depend on fetal activity or position are as reliable as any other sex-determination myth—about 50 percent of the time (which is just enough to keep the belief going).

FACT OR FICTION?

"Don't raise your arms above your head while you're pregnant; it will make the baby's cord wrap around his neck."

This is probably the most common and widespread myth about pregnancy. But, don't worry. There's no connection between your arm muscles and your baby's cord. When a cord does get wrapped around a baby, it's usually caused by the baby's own movements. About 25 percent of all babies are born with the cord wrapped around the neck. In most cases, it's not a problem. But, if the cord is very short or the baby is very big, it can cause trouble. That's why it's so important that your baby be delivered by an experienced and skilled birth attendant in whom you have confidence.

COMFORT

What to Do

❑ Do Super-Dooper Arm Reaches (below), a variation of the Arm Reaches on page 59, to stimulate blood flow to and from your hands.

❑ Give yourself a Finger Massage (below).

EXERCISE TECHNIQUES

SUPER-DOOPER ARM REACHES

Benefits: Relieves temporary numbness, tingling, or swelling in the fingers, relieves shortness of breath, reduces tension and fatigue, and energizes.

1. Sit or stand in a comfortable position with your arms at your sides.
2. Inhale as you raise one arm high over your head, stretching from the waist. (Don't let your hip or foot rise.)
3. While your hand is still in the air, wiggle your fingers, as though you're playing a piano.
4. Exhale as you pull your arm back down to your side.
5. Repeat with the other arm.
6. Repeat several times.
7. Follow by vigorously shaking both hands.

MASSAGE TECHNIQUES

FINGER MASSAGE

Benefits: Relieves temporary numbness, swelling, tingling, or stiffness in the fingers.

1. Beginning with the small finger of one hand, use the other hand to gently but firmly push the finger back as far as you comfortably can. (Don't worry if your knuckles pop. This harmless popping is just tiny bubbles in the fluid around the joint. And it won't make your knuckles get bigger, despite what they told you when you were a kid.)
2. One at a time, push each finger and then the thumb, holding the pressure for a few seconds each time.
3. When you finish one hand, continue with the other.
4. After doing both hands, go back to the small finger of the first hand.
5. Use the thumb and first two fingers of the second hand to stroke

firmly downward from the nail of the small finger to the base, as if you were trying to put on a pair of tight gloves. (This feels better if you first apply a small amount of lotion to your fingers.)

6. Slowly repeat this stroking three times on each finger.

(*See also* Swelling, page 108.)

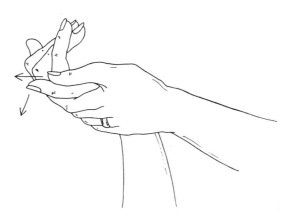

Finger Massage—Steps 1-3

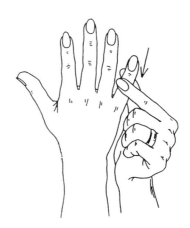

Finger Massage—Steps 4-6

Gas

Increased intestinal gas is a common and sometimes embarrassing side effect of pregnancy. It's caused in part by the weight of your growing baby pressing on your intestines, forcing them to move more slowly. The problem is compounded by the hormonal changes taking place in your body, which also slow down intestinal movement. Gas may be unpleasant and it can sometimes be embarrassing, but it's simply the natural result of food spending more time in your intestines.

PREVENTION

What to Avoid

❏ Avoid the usual gas-formers, such as beans, strong-flavored greens, and spices. It's impossible to prevent some intestinal gas from forming, whether or not you are pregnant. But you may find that foods that never bothered you before now cause you to form gas, so watch your diet to see if there's a relationship between certain foods and an increased amount of gas.

COMFORT

What to Do

❑ Stimulate your intestines by starting each day with a warm drink. An excellent one is a glass of hot water with the juice of half a lemon.

❑ Exercise regularly. Walking or swimming several times each week can help your body eliminate gas. Other exercises that encourage the release of excess gas are the Pelvic Tilt (page 10), the Buttocks Curl (page 11), and the Knee-Chest position (page 7).

What to Avoid

❑ Avoid anti-gas medications without consulting your birth attendant.

(*See also* Constipation, page 36.)

Groin Pain

WHEN IT'S MORE THAN JUST A PAIN

Be careful not to confuse this harmless, occasional groin pain with the persistent pain that comes with an ectopic pregnancy, appendicitis, and other emergency conditions. Notify your health professional if the pain lasts longer than two minutes or if it's accompanied by weakness, headache, shoulder pain, nausea, dizziness, cramping, or bleeding.

During the first month or two you were pregnant, you may have felt a sudden twinge in or near your groin. This pain is usually caused by a spasm of the fallopian tube, and is a normal occurrence. Later, in the second and third trimester, you may notice a sudden, sharp pain that starts in your groin and shoots up the side of your abdomen. It may happen when you first get out of bed in the morning, or when you do something that involves twisting at the waist, or even when you sneeze. This time the pain comes from a spasm of one of the round ligaments that hold your uterus in place. Ordinarily these ligaments are quite short, but during pregnancy they have to stretch to keep up with your growing uterus. The stretching leaves them irritable and sensitive so that they cramp easily if you make a sudden or twisting movement.

PREVENTION

What to Do

❑ Move slowly when turning in bed or getting out of bed. Instead of turning from your back by first moving your legs and then your torso, use a log-roll motion to move your entire body at the same time.

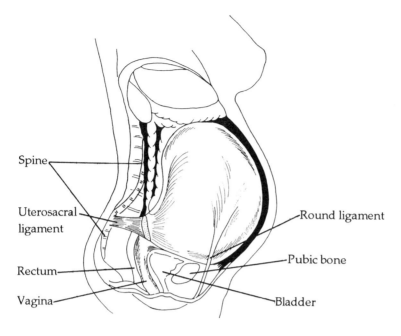

Spine

Uterosacral
ligament

Round ligament

Rectum

Pubic bone

Vagina

Bladder

Uterine Ligaments

What to Avoid

❑ Avoid sudden or jerking movements, especially those that require you to twist or turn at the waist.

COMFORT

What to Do

❑ Bend at the waist toward the side that hurts. This should let the ligament relax and should relieve the pain. *Notify your doctor or midwife if the pain lasts longer than two minutes.*

Gum Bleeding

The hormonal changes you're going through affect the mucous membranes in your body, including the gums. As a result, you may notice that your gums are sensitive and swollen, and that they sometimes bleed when you brush your teeth.

PREVENTION

What to Do

- ☐ Eat one or two good sources of vitamin C daily. This nutrient helps strengthen and repair body cells and is found in citrus fruits, broccoli, potatoes, tomatoes, and other fruits and vegetables. (The Recommended Daily Requirement of vitamin C during pregnancy is 80 milligrams. If you take a vitamin C supplement, do not take more than 1,000 milligrams daily.)
- ☐ Use a soft toothbrush to clean your teeth and gums after every meal. Follow this by flossing.
- ☐ If increased sensitivity makes it hard to clean your gums, ask your dentist to check them for you. (Be sure to tell him you're pregnant and that you want to avoid dental x-rays.)

COMFORT

What to Do

- ☐ See Prevention tips.

Hair Changes

FACT OR FICTION?

A permanent won't "take" when you're pregnant.

Contrary to myth, pregnancy does not affect the results you get from a permanent. On the other hand, hair care products are among the multitude of substances that have not been tested sufficiently to determine whether they're safe to use during pregnancy. We don't have proof that they're bad for you or your baby, but we don't have proof that they aren't, so you may want to hold off on a permanent or dye job, at least until after the first trimester.

As pregnancy changes your shape, you may begin to feel more concerned than usual about the rest of your appearance. While there's not much you can do about your shape, there are several things you can do about your hair.

Throughout most of your life, the individual hairs rotate through phases, with some growing, some resting, and some falling. During pregnancy, these phases are interrupted by hormonal changes, leaving more hairs in a resting phase. As a result, your hair may be thicker than usual. (The bad news is that after your baby is born, all those hairs that didn't fall out during pregnancy will do so, leaving your hair a bit thinner than normal for a month or two.)

Your hair is also affected by your diet. Hair stylists comment that they notice an improvement in the body and lustre of the expectant mother's hair after she begins taking prenatal vitamins. Some expectant mothers find that the vitamins seem to make their hair grow faster, too.

COMFORT

What to Do

- ❏ Use a gentle brush, such as one made of boar's hair bristles or a plastic brush used for blow-dry styling.
- ❏ Increase the amount of conditioning you usually give your hair.
- ❏ Ask a professional hair stylist to recommend a hairstyle and a conditioning program that will make your hair easier to care for now, as well as after the baby comes.

What to Avoid

- ❏ Avoid overworking your hair. Too much brushing or too much heat can damage it.

Headaches

The hormonal changes of pregnancy can affect the number and frequency of headaches you experience. Some women have fewer headaches when they're pregnant, while others have more. The most common headaches fall into two categories, migraine and tension headaches.

Migraine Headaches

A migraine headache causes intense throbbing that's usually limited to one side of the head. (The word "migraine" comes from a word meaning "half a head," but the pain can affect both sides.) Some people experience a warning sensation, called an *aura*, before the onset of pain. This might be a visual or an auditory disturbance or an odd smell, or you might just know a migraine is coming because you always feel a certain undefinable way beforehand. Other symptoms of migraine include nausea, dizziness, and sensitivity to light, noise, and sudden movement. (When I have a migraine, all I want to do is hide in bed with all the lights off and the blankets pulled over my head.)

There are a number of theories as to what causes migraines, but the most commonly accepted is that the attack is caused by vaso-constriction—a temporary narrowing of the blood vessels in the brain. When your brain doesn't get enough blood, it responds by dilating, or widening, the blood vessels. This greatly increases the blood flow in the brain, and it's thought that this oversupply of blood causes the pain.

PREVENTION

What to Do

❑ Exercise regularly. Physical activity, such as walking, biking, or swimming, aids circulation, improves energy, reduces fatigue, and increases your sense of well-being.

What to Avoid

❑ Avoid substances that may trigger a migraine in a susceptible individual. The worst culprits are chocolate, caffeine drinks, red wines, red meats, strong cheeses, and some preserved meats.
❑ Avoid skipping meals, especially during stressful times.
❑ Avoid situations that may trigger a migraine. Two common ones are glaring sunlight and insufficient sleep.
❑ Avoid all triggers, especially when you're under stress or when a stressful situation has just passed. Although migraines are not emotional in origin, emotional strain does make your body more susceptible to an attack either during or just after the upsetting situation.

COMFORT

What to Do

❑ As soon as you feel a migraine coming on, seek out a dark, quiet place where you can close your eyes and rest.
❑ Apply an ice pack to the back of your head to encourage a decrease in blood flow.
❑ Use the Temple Massage. (See page 69.)
❑ Use the Upper Neck Massage. (See page 69.)
❑ Because the problem of migraine is one of blood flow, you may be able to relieve it by learning to control the movement of your blood. This is something patients learn in biofeedback clinics, but you can

learn it at home. During an attack, the temperature of your hands usually drops, probably due to decreased blood flow in your arms and legs as more blood is drawn to the brain. Try the Hand Warming technique on page 71 to redirect the blood flow away from your brain and back toward your limbs.

❏ Place an ice pack on the point of pain, or on one of the pressure points shown in this section. A good way to find the right point is to apply pressure to each. The point or points that feel very sore and tender are the ones that need attention. Either you or a partner can stimulate these points with your thumb or fingers before applying ice. The stimulation increases the effectiveness of the treatment.

What to Avoid

❏ Do not apply moist or dry heat to your head during a migraine.

❏ Avoid taking aspirin, ibuprofen, or other medications. If you absolutely must take something, use an aspirin substitute. Do not exceed the recommended daily dosage and do not take it for more than two days without consulting your birth attendant.

Tension Headaches

With the many physical and emotional changes you are undergoing now, you may be having more than your share of tension headaches. These are characterized by a feeling of tightness in the head or neck, as though someone placed a metal band around your head.

PREVENTION

What to Do

❏ Examine any emotional causes of tension. You and your family are dealing with new pressures now. Pregnancy involves many short- and long-term changes in your lives. Talk about your goals and concerns. Decide together which things you want to change and what you can do to achieve these changes.

❏ Examine any physical sources of muscular tension. This may be connected with an emotional concern, or it may be totally physical in origin. For example, when you drive, do you allow your shoulders to rest comfortably low, or do you hold them up, close to your ears? Drop them and feel how much more relaxed you are. When reading, thinking, or listening to someone else, what do you do with your lower jaw? Many people find that they tighten it without realizing. Let go and you'll feel your neck relax and your shoulders loosen. Of course, you don't have to go around with your mouth hanging open. You can close your mouth and then let your jaw drop slightly to relax it.

What to Avoid

❑ Avoid stressful situations whenever possible. If you can't avoid them, face them with a supportive partner or friend.
❑ Avoid unrealistic expectations of yourself, your partner, and your pregnancy.

COMFORT

What to Do

❑ Use the Shoulder Massage. (See page 22.)
❑ Use the Facial Massage. (See page 70.)
❑ Use the Soothing Touch Massage. (See page 69.)
❑ Use Sequential Relaxation. (See page 72.)
❑ Use the Relaxation Countdown. (See page 73.)
❑ Try a soothing cup of herbal tea or a glass of milk.

What to Avoid

❑ Avoid as much stress as possible while you have a tension headache.
❑ Avoid taking aspirin, ibuprofen, and most other medications. If you absolutely must take something, make it an aspirin substitute. Do not exceed the recommended dosage, and do not take it for more than two days without consulting your birth attendant.

MASSAGE TECHNIQUES

Before trying these massage techniques, it's a good idea to review the information on massage in the section called "How to Use This Book." Each individual responds differently to massage, so feel free to make changes in the pattern and intensity of pressure, *as long as the recipient is comfortable with the changes.*

Most of the pressure patterns described in this section can be used for any of the massage techniques.

TEMPLE MASSAGE

Benefits: Relieves headache or tension and relaxes.

1. Place your first two fingers at the indentation of your temples, just below the pulse. (See figure on this page.)
2. Use thumbs or fingers to apply firm, gentle pressure, moving in a slow, circular pattern that draws the skin across the bone.

UPPER NECK MASSAGE

Benefits: Relaxes and relieves headache, especially migraine or tension headache. (To relieve nausea, apply pressure or ice.)

1. Place your thumbs at the back of the head, just below the skull and directly over the neck bones, or cervical spine. (If you bend your head back, you should feel a ridge of muscle just outside each thumb. See figure on this page.)
2. Now, slide your thumbs out toward the sides, until they're just outside the ridge of muscle, where it makes a corner with the skull bone.
3. Let your head drop forward and push your thumbs up into the corner and press firmly for sixty seconds.
4. Slide your thumbs out farther, until just behind and under the ridge of bone behind each ear (mastoid process).
5. Push your thumbs up toward the bone and press firmly for sixty seconds.
6. Repeat for thirty to sixty seconds, three times on each point.
7. Finish with a firm, kneading massage to the entire area.

Comments: For relief of nausea that accompanies migraine, apply pressure or ice to the points just behind the mastoid process.

SOOTHING TOUCH

Benefits: Relaxes, and restores a sense of calm and control.

1. Place your fingers near the top of your forehead, where the natural hairline is usually located.
2. Slowly slide your fingers back and forth near the midline until you feel a shallow indentation where the bone barely protrudes on

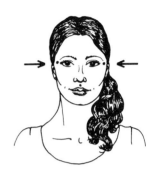

Pressure Points for Temple Massage

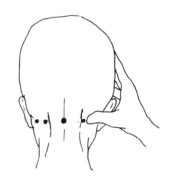

Pressure Points for Upper Neck Massage

either side. These protrusions are called the *frontal prominences.*

3. Lay your fingers across this area, as though you were resting your head in your hand.

4. Close your eyes and breathe in a slow, relaxed manner. Just resting your hand here is often enough, but you may also apply gentle, steady pressure or move your fingers back and forth across your forehead, slowly moving the skin across the bone as the sensation of calmness and control washes over you.

LABOR TIPS

The Soothing Touch is great for helping control anxiety or panic during labor. If you or your partner starts to feel anxious or panicky during labor, place your hand across your forehead, close your eyes, and take several slow, deep breaths. Focus on letting the sensation of calm and control wash over you, flowing from your head down through your body.

FACIAL MASSAGE

Benefits: Relaxes and relieves headache, and reduces tension and fatigue.

(This one works best when done by your partner. For that reason, the directions are written for him or her.)

1. Stand or sit behind your partner and place your thumbs on top of her head and the first two fingers of each hand over the frontal prominences (see Soothing Touch, above).

2. Pull your fingers slowly and firmly across the forehead, moving out and down toward the temples. (See figure on this page.)

3. As you reach the temples, do a slow, circular massage on each side. (Spend as much time massaging the temples as you did moving toward them.)

4. Move your fingers back to the starting point and repeat as many times as desired. Remember, keep it slow and rhythmic, and keep your thumbs in contact with her head so that her concentration isn't broken.

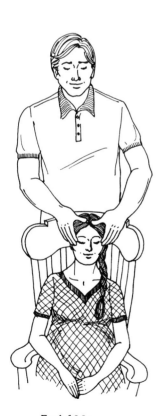

Facial Massage

Comments: This massage is far more relaxing and effective if you both inhale as the fingers move out toward the temples and exhale as they circle the temples. Remember, keep it slow and easy.

Facial massage feels so good that you and your partner may want to take turns doing it to each other every night. If you are giving the treatment, you may sit on the floor or bed and have your partner lay his head in your lap, or you may sit or stand behind your seated partner.

RELAXATION TECHNIQUES

HAND WARMING

Benefits: Relaxes, and helps relieve pain.

(This works best if you tape the instructions to play while you relax, or if someone slowly and quietly reads them aloud, pausing between each step.)

1. Get into a comfortable position, making sure all your body parts are well-supported on pillows.
2. Close your eyes and sigh deeply.
3. Start breathing slowly and easily.
4. As you inhale, note the coolness of the air entering your body.
5. As you exhale, note the warmth.
6. The cool inhalation brings energy into your body, the warm exhalation sends tension out of your body as relaxation spreads throughout your being.
7. Continue breathing slowly and feel the cool and warm intervals.
8. Now let the inhalations happen automatically. Don't pay attention to them. Note only the warm exhalations.
9. As you exhale, let the air flow through your arms and into the palms of your hands, spreading warmth throughout the hand.
10. Lie still and let the exhalation flow into your palms and through the fingertips, leaving your hands heavy, warm, and limp.
11. Notice the palms begin to tingle as they fill with warmth.
12. Rest a while and focus on the feeling of warmth and tingling in your hands as they lay limp and heavy on the pillow or bed.

If this exercise was difficult for you, try doing it one hand at a time. If you still don't feel the warmth, sit with your hands on your lap. Shake one hand vigorously and let it drop to your lap. Note the difference in your two hands. The one you shook is warm and you can feel the blood moving through it. This is the sensation you want to achieve. As you do the relaxation, imagine the blood flowing through each cell of your hand, bringing oxygen, warmth, and relaxation. You can help yourself achieve the warmth by practicing a while with your hands in warm water or with a heating pad on a low setting. After a bit of practice, you won't need the props. You'll imagine warm water flowing over your hand, as in a whirlpool bath, and you'll feel the warmth spread through your hands.

SEQUENTIAL RELAXATION

1. Close your eyes and sigh deeply. Begin inhaling through your nose to a slow count of four, and exhaling through your mouth to a slow count of four. Continue breathing in this manner throughout the session.
2. Roll your head gently from side to side and let it come to rest in the middle.
3. Inhale through the nose to a count of four. Exhale through the mouth to a count of four.
4. Let your jaw drop slightly.
5. Squeeze your shoulder blades together behind you.
6. Release your shoulders and let your arms flop heavily onto the bed (or chair), resting with the palms facing upward, the fingers slightly curled.
7. Continue breathing in through the nose to a count of four and out through the mouth to a count of four.
8. Press your lower back into the bed.
9. Release your back and let your legs rest and your feet flop outward.
10. Now go back through your body from your head to your toes and feel relaxation in each part.
11. Feel relaxation in your face, jaw, and neck.
12. Feel the loose, heavy feeling in your shoulders, arms, and hands.
13. Feel the soft fullness of your abdomen as it relaxes.
14. Feel the heaviness and warmth of your buttocks, thighs, legs, and feet.
15. In through the nose, out through the mouth.
16. Go back to your forehead. Feel the relaxation. Let it feel as though your eyes are heavy and your lids are drooping.
17. Let your cheeks feel warm and full. Feel the release in your lower jaw.
18. Each time you exhale, let your shoulders and back sink into the bed.
19. With each exhalation let your back get longer and looser.
20. Let your buttocks and thighs melt and mold to the shape of the mattress.
21. As you exhale, feel your legs getting heavy and warm and melting into the bed.
22. Sigh deeply as you experience the release and relaxation of your entire body.

By progressing from one end of your body to another, you can achieve a sense of total release. If you're having trouble learning to relax, try some of these tips from my classes:

❑ As you practice each relaxation exercise, note which words signal your body to relax. Use those that help and ignore the rest.

❑ If the four-count is too fast or slow, set a more comfortable pace by changing the number.

❑ If counting just doesn't work for you, forget about it and focus on something else. I often use a Bible verse as a focal point. I find one that has an even number of syllables, and then divide the phrase into two parts, inhaling on one and exhaling on the second. For example:

Inhale { Be Still And Know   Exhale { That I Am God

Sometimes a song works better:

Inhale { Rock- A- Bye Baby   Exhale { In The Tree Top   Inhale { When The Wind Blows   Exhale { The Cradle Will Rock

(With a song, follow the beat and rhythm of the music instead of the syllables.)

❑ If the idea of warmth and heaviness was most effective for you, use these words and feelings to relax. If you could feel the release more strongly when you exhaled as you let go of a muscle, concentrate on this.

RELAXATION COUNTDOWN

Benefits: Relaxes, and helps relieve pain.

1. Close your eyes and take a deep sigh.
2. Take a slow, deep inhalation, followed by a slow, deep exhalation. Continue breathing in this manner, maintaining a slow, steady rhythm.
3. As you breathe, start counting silently (or ask your partner to count)

from one to ten, letting each number fall during an exhalation. (Inhale/Out one, Inhale/Out two, Inhale/Out three, etc.)

4. With each number and each exhalation, let your body get looser, limper, and more relaxed. When you reach the number ten, sigh and remain at rest for a while. (If you achieve profound relaxation, slowly bring yourself out of it by reversing the countdown.)

Heartburn

Heartburn is a term used to describe a burning or painful sensation in the stomach. We call it heartburn because the discomfort is most noticeable at the upper end of the stomach, which is located near your heart. (I've always found it interesting that we call a pain in the stomach "heartburn," but a pain in the intestine is a "stomach-ache.")

One of the most common complaints of pregnancy, heartburn is caused by the crowded conditions inside your abdomen and by increased stomach acid due to hormonal changes. The problem is especially pronounced in the last months of pregnancy. You may not be able to eat as much as before, and you may feel short of breath after you do eat. But perhaps the worst part of heartburn is the recurring experience of waking up at night with a sudden sensation of burning acid in the throat. This happens when the narrow, upper portion of the stomach is pushed up into the opening in your diaphragm so that part of it rests in the chest cavity. This condition is called a *functional hiatal hernia* or *diaphragmatic hernia*. It sounds awful, but it usually corrects itself as soon as the baby drops low enough to let the stomach move back down where it belongs. If not, it probably will improve after the birth.

PREVENTION

What to Do

❑ Sleep in a semi-sitting position. If you notice more heartburn at night, it may have something to do with your sleeping position. Turn back to page 5 and look at the figure. Now, imagine what would happen if this woman were to lie on her back—her baby would fall toward her stomach, placing even more pressure on it. To avoid this situation, simply sleep with several pillows propped under your head and upper torso.

❑ Eat smaller, more frequent meals to allow for the decreased amount of room in your stomach.

What to Avoid

❑ Avoid spicy foods, as well as any that seem to increase your indigestion. (Take heart—you'll probably be able to eat all your favorites again as soon as the baby is born.)

❑ Avoid eating just before going to bed.

COMFORT

What to Do

❑ Use the Knee-Chest position. I know it looks as if this position, which places your head lower than your hips, would only make things worse, but it doesn't. It seems to ease indigestion by taking pressure off of the stomach and intestines. (I didn't believe it either, but after teaching over 5,000 pregnant women, I'm forced to accept the fact that it works.)

❑ Use the Super-Dooper Arm Reaches on page 60. No one is quite sure why, but it may be that this action helps the stomach to recede toward the abdominal cavity. If you have frequent bouts with indigestion, do these reaches about fifteen minutes before and after each meal.

What to Avoid

❑ Avoid commercial antacids made with anything other than calcium. Calcium is nature's own antacid. It actually neutralizes excess sto-mach acid and helps the digestive system function more efficiently. Calcium is also available in milk products, such as cheese, yogurt, ice cream, and milk. If you don't like these foods, or if you're allergic to them, ask your pharmacist for calcium tablets or liquid. Follow the directions, keeping your total calcium intake, including that from foods, to about 1,200 milligrams a day. Remember, too much calcium can cause leg cramps and other problems.

(*See also* Constipation, page 36; and Gas, page 61.)

Hemorrhoids

As your pregnancy progresses, the pressure on your pelvic region increases, making it more difficult for blood to flow freely in and out of the area. At the same time, the increased amount of fluid in your blood stream slows the circulation even further. As a result of this pressure and strain on the blood vessels, you may develop hemorrhoids, or piles. These are enlarged veins, similar to the varicose veins some women develop in their legs. Hemorrhoids may be internal, or they may protrude through the rectal opening, or anus. (An external hemorrhoid feels like a soft lump or bulge at the anus.) Hemorrhoids may cause bleeding, itching, and pain, or they may cause no symptoms at all.

There's a familial tendency toward weak blood vessels, so if one or both of your parents have hemorrhoids or varicose veins, you're more likely to develop them, too.

PREVENTION

What to Do

❑ Drink lots of fluids and eat whole grains and raw fruits and vegetables. This will help prevent constipation and reduce your risk of developing hemorrhoids. (Refer to page 36 for more information on constipation.)

What to Avoid

❑ Avoid constipation. Straining to have a bowel movement puts pressure on pelvic blood vessels, which increases your chances of developing hemorrhoids.

COMFORT

What to Do

❑ Practice the Kegel exercise (page 28) frequently throughout each day to encourage a good blood flow to and from your pelvic area.
❑ For temporary relief of pain, sit in a tub of very warm water.
❑ When trying to have a bowel movement, place your feet on a small stool or box. This will provide better leverage and help avoid over-straining.
❑ To reduce swelling and discomfort, elevate your hips by using the Knee-Chest position (page 7) or by lying on your back and placing pillows under your hips. While in this inverted position, apply cotton balls soaked in cold witch hazel to your rectum. The witch hazel will help shrink the hemorrhoids, and the inverted posture will encourage the excess blood to start circulating more efficiently.

❏ Check with your own physician or midwife before using any commercial hemorrhoid preparations.

Caution: If you have bleeding or severe pain, consult your physician or midwife.

(*See also* Constipation, page 36; Pelvic Pressure, page 96; and Varicose Veins, page 112.)

Hip Pain

As your baby grows, he exerts pressure on nerves and joints that aren't accustomed to that much extra weight. At the same time, a hormone called *relaxin* begins to soften the cartilage in your hip joints to allow the bones to spread slightly, making more room for the baby. These changes give you an unstable base of support for the added weight. As a result of these changes, you may experience twinges, cramps, or even charley horses in the buttocks, hips, and thighs.

Some women have more severe pain because their sacroiliac joint, which joins the back of the pelvis to the tailbone, has relaxed and is pressing on the sacroiliac nerve. This can cause a sharp, shooting pain that runs down the back of the leg.

When I was eight-plus months pregnant, my right hip locked on me a couple of times. It didn't hurt, but I couldn't move my leg until whatever was wrong had righted itself. By that time I was spending most of the day at home anyway, so it usually wasn't a problem. But I'll never forget the afternoon I carried a bag of trash out to the apartment dumpster only to have my hip lock before I could get back to our door. I lay there on the sidewalk for a few minutes, feeling like a fool, until a man came and started staring at me. Then, while this strong young man watched, I did a combination leg-drag and crawl for about 100 yards. My hip unlocked just as I reached our apartment, so I got up, hurried inside, and slammed the door, leaving my observer to wonder what in the world he had witnessed.

PREVENTION

What to Avoid

❏ Avoid carrying heavy objects.
❏ Avoid high-impact aerobics and other exercises that put added strain or weight on your hips or knees.

COMFORT

What to Do

- ❑ Use the Bridge (page 7).
- ❑ Use the Knee-Chest position (page 7).
- ❑ Use the Kneeling Pelvic Tilt (page 19).
- ❑ Use the Buttocks Curl (page 11).
- ❑ Use Knee-Rocking (below).
- ❑ Use Lower Back Massage (below), or apply heat or ice to these lower back pressure points.
- ❑ Apply heat or ice over your tailbone.

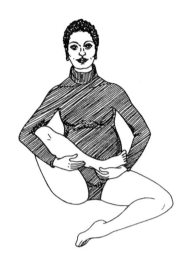

Knee-Rocking

EXERCISE TECHNIQUES

KNEE-ROCKING

Benefits: Stretches ligaments in the hip joint to ease tension and pressure on them, stimulates a better blood supply to the nerves in the hip area, and feels good.

1. Sit on the floor or bed with one leg either extended or folded in front of you.
2. Use both arms to lift the other leg, bending it at the knee and bringing it toward your chest and abdomen. (See figure on this page.)
3. Straighten your back and cradle your leg in your arms, holding it as high and as close to you as is possible without straining.
4. Moving from the hip joint, gently rock the leg back and forth, as though you were rocking your baby.
5. After rocking one leg several times, switch to the other leg.

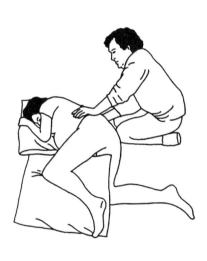

Lower Back Massage

MASSAGE TECHNIQUES

LOWER BACK MASSAGE

Benefits: Relieves pain and tension in lower back, and reduces fatigue.

1. Place your hands on your waist with your fingers pointed toward your spine.
2. Slide your hands toward the center of your back until you can feel the groove on either side of the backbone. (See figure on this page.)
3. Apply firm, steady pressure on both sides for several minutes. (Heat or cold may be substituted.)

Indigestion

See Gas; Heartburn.

Insomnia

Sleep patterns vary throughout pregnancy. For the first three months or so, you may feel overwhelmingly tired and may find it takes a great deal of energy just to stay awake past nine or ten in the evening. Although the fatigue usually lifts during the second trimester, it often returns by the seventh or eighth month when the added weight and stress of pregnancy are reaching a peak. Ironically, other pregnancy-related changes may keep you from sleeping, even when you're tired. You may have to get up several times a night to go to the bathroom. Then, once you get back to bed, you may lie awake worrying whether your baby will be a healthy one or your labor a difficult one. And when you finally do fall asleep, your rest may be disturbed by unpleasant dreams. In the end, even if you manage to get eight hours of sleep, all these stresses and interruptions can rob you of any real rest. Fortunately, there are several ways to help yourself.

PREVENTION

What to Do

❑ Try to identify sources of tension and take positive steps toward eliminating or reducing them. Remember that you were created as a mental, physical, and spiritual being, and that each aspect of your being responds to disturbances in the others. Talk with your spouse about any concerns or fears you may have regarding the upcoming birth, how a baby will change your life or your marriage, finances, or other areas of your life, and work together to resolve them. If you're concerned about the birth, talk with your birth attendant and enroll in childbirth education classes so you'll be ready to deal with the ups and downs of labor. Just getting started toward finding a solution will give you a sense of peace.

❑ Choose sleep positions that are truly comfortable. This may require a different sleeping system as the shape of your body changes. Try placing pillows in various places until you're well supported and relaxed. If you're lying on your back, place an extra pillow or a wedge-shaped cushion behind you to reduce heartburn and short-ness of breath. A pillow under your thighs will help relax your back and legs. When you rest on your side, try a pillow between your legs. Later, as your baby grows and your abdomen pulls toward the bed, tuck a small pillow or rolled towel underneath it.

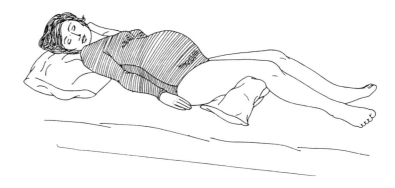

Back-Lying Position

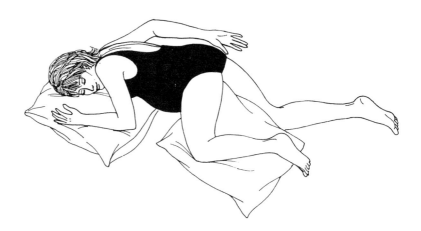

Side-Lying Position

❑ Establish a bedtime routine. When parents ask how to get a fussy child to sleep at night, they're usually told to establish a routine and to stick to it. This advice works for adults, too. You may already have a routine of sorts. You probably get undressed, brush your teeth, and wash your face in the same order each night. Once in bed, you might pray or read or watch television or listen to music until you feel sleepy. After years of doing it this way, these simple rituals signal your body and mind that it's time to sleep.

What to Avoid

❏ Avoid vigorous exercise within two hours of your usual bedtime.
❏ Avoid exposure to stressful situations just before bedtime.
❏ Avoid caffeine products as much as possible.
❏ Avoid eating a heavy or spicy meal within two hours of your usual bedtime.

COMFORT

What to Do

❏ Drink milk (warm or cold) before going to bed. Milk contains a natural element called *tryptophan* that helps induce relaxation.
❏ Drink a cup of chamomile or lemon tea with a little honey before bedtime.
❏ Eat a small bedtime snack, something that's high in carbohydrates, such as a cookie or cracker.
❏ Use the Soothing Touch (page 69) and Facial Massage (page 70).
❏ Use the Relaxation Countdown (page 73).
❏ Use Sequential Relaxation (page 72).
❏ Use The Swing relaxation technique (page 82).
❏ Take a warm bath before trying to sleep. Be sure the water is not hot—just warm. Too much heat over your entire body will tire you, but warmth will relax you. You might also want to bring along your milk or tea and dim the lights. Just remember not to fall asleep in the tub. When you start feeling drowsy, get out slowly and pat yourself dry with a soft towel. Then climb into bed and snuggle down into the sheets and sleep.

What to Avoid

❏ Do not take any type of sleep medication during pregnancy. Some may harm your baby, and many can cause you to become dependent on them.

RELAXATION TECHNIQUES

THE SWING

Benefits: Induces relaxation, and provides a focal point for use in labor.

1. Close your eyes and sigh deeply.
2. Begin breathing slowly and easily.
3. As you continue breathing slowly and easily, imagine a swing gently swaying back and forth.
4. Inhale, letting your breath pull the swing toward you.
5. Exhale, letting your breath gently push the swing away.
6. Keep the rhythm slow and easy, moving the swing back and forth as you breathe.
7. As you continue to breathe the swing back and forth, your breaths begin to slow and the swing begins to slow. Each time your exhalation gently pushes away the swing, it leaves you feeling limp and loose and relaxed.

Comments: Before trying The Swing, turn back to page xvii-xix and review the information on the use of sight, sound, and sensation in relaxing. Then, as you practice The Swing, focus on the sensory details that work for you. For example, a sight person might watch the swing, while a sensation person might feel the motion as it sways back and forth.

Keep in mind that each person relaxes in her own way. If you're uncomfortable with the swing moving toward you when you inhale, let it move side to side. And if a swing just doesn't work for you, imagine a swinging pendulum or a small sailboat floating back and forth on a lake.

(*See also* Mood Changes, page 83.)

Joint Pain

Although arthritis patients sometimes have less pain during pregnancy, some women who've never had problems before experience frequent aching in their joints. This may be due to the extra weight the joints have to support during pregnancy, or to the increased fluid in the tissues. Whatever its cause, these women usually report that their symptoms disappear after giving birth.

Mood Changes 83

COMFORT

What to Do

- ❏ Use the finger exercises on page 60 and 61 for pain in hand and finger joints.
- ❏ Use Knee-Rocking (page 78) and the Leg Stretch (page 45) for pain in the hips or knees.
- ❏ Apply a kneading massage to aching hands, arms, feet, or knees. (*Do not massage your thighs or calves.*)
- ❏ When a massage is not possible, you may be able to reduce some joint pain by lightly scratching the skin over the painful area.
- ❏ Apply a heating pad or hot water bottle to painful joints.
- ❏ Soak in a warm bath. If you prefer a shower, place a plastic stool on the shower floor so you can sit under the stream of water. Whether you bathe or shower, do not use very hot water. It may not be good for your baby, and can leave you feeling dizzy and fatigued, as well.

What to Avoid

- ❏ *Avoid massaging your thighs or calves with a kneading action or deep pressure during pregnancy or postpartum.* Blood clots are more common in these areas during pregnancy and postpartum. If a clot has developed, a deep, kneading massage could disturb it, allowing it to enter the bloodstream where it could cause serious complications.
- ❏ *Do not take aspirin or ibuprofen during pregnancy.* These drugs can increase the risk of bleeding for you and your baby. If you need medication, ask your doctor about taking an aspirin substitute. If he says you may, be careful to take it only occasionally, and not on a regular basis.

Mood Changes

"It seems like the longer my wife is pregnant, the more sensitive she gets."

"Moods. I hate my moods."

"I can't keep from crying at little things. My poor husband is so confused he doesn't know what to say to me anymore. I'm surprised we talk at all."

Both men and women may experience mood swings during pregnancy. This is a normal reaction to the many changes taking place in your lives. You may feel happy and excited one day as you plan for your baby's arrival and dream of the time when you'll hold him in your arms. But then, the next day, depression may set in as you wonder whether you made the right decision about having a baby. Sometimes it seems as if you've been pregnant forever, and you think the world will come to an end before your pregnancy does. At other times you feel fulfilled and privileged—like a link in the chain of human history.

There are many reasons for all these different feelings. Sometimes you can point to a physical cause. For example, you may be shopping happily for maternity clothes when you catch a glimpse of yourself in a shop window or mirror and realize how much and how quickly your body has changed. Suddenly you feel depressed and lose all interest in shopping. Or you and your husband may have been looking forward to going to a party, but as the evening approaches, fatigue sets in and all you want to do is go to bed. As you lie there in the dark, you realize this is not typical for you, and you begin to grieve for the memory of how things used to be, before you were pregnant. These changes in your mood and outlook are direct results of the physical realities of pregnancy. Fortunately, as you can see in this book, most of them can be handled and minimized. Even those that cannot be overcome are easier to accept if you understand their causes and if you remember that they are temporary.

What about the mood changes that seem to have no physical origin? Some of these are the result of how you and your partner and those around you react to the pregnancy and the changes in your lives. If you're working outside the home, your spouse may feel bad about not providing the family's full support. If you're not working, *you* may feel bad about the added financial burden on him. In this time of population control, friends sometimes react negatively to the second, third, or fourth child. They may insinuate that you should have waited or make jokes about your "accident." This can make you feel angry or guilty or both. Your relationship with your parents may change, too. You may feel closer to them than ever before, or you may feel estranged.

Men often comment that their wives seem more sensitive when pregnant. They cry more, and it seems difficult to say the right thing to them. "The Hormonal Theory" and "The New Awareness Theory" are possible explanations of this (see inset). Or maybe, as one of my friends suggested, the unpredictability of feelings and of pregnancy itself is God's way of preparing you for the unpredictability of parenthood.

Two Theories
Regarding Mood Changes

The Hormonal Theory. During pregnancy your body produces a high level of the hormone progesterone. This same hormone is at a high level just before the onset of menstruation, when many women suffer from the premenstrual syndrome (PMS) that causes tension, moodiness, and irritability. Many experts blame progesterone for causing similar problems in pregnancy. It's like waiting nine months for your period to start, but it never does.

The New Awareness Theory. Another explanation for the extra sensitivity pregnant women often feel lies in the many new sensations and changes occurring within your body. Ordinarily we shut out the normal physical sensations of our body's daily activities. We don't notice the peristaltic movements as our intestines digest food and move it along the way. We barely pay heed to the heart as it beats, sending blood pulsating and coursing through every cell in the body. Normal inhalations and exhalations pass barely noticed. But now, you feel dozens of new physical sensations. You can feel, and perhaps even see, the pulsating of your uterine artery. And you can't miss the sloshing of amniotic fluid as your baby kicks and rolls about inside you. Each new sensation demands your attention. You stop and notice how it feels and you try to imagine that you can see inside your womb and watch your baby growing and moving. As you begin to pay more attention to these new sensations, you notice old ones as well. The intestinal movements feel a lot like the first flutters your baby makes. Even indigestion and constipation take on new meanings as you wonder how your own health affects your baby. Every sensation seems newly significant.

This new focus on everyday occurrences can extend to the outside world as you look at people and events with new awareness. You evaluate everything that is said, turning it over several times to find out what it really means. This is simply an extension of your concern for what's going on within your body, but it can be a problem because you may find a meaning that was not intended. Just as that twinge in your side is probably a tense ligament and not a danger sign, what seems like an insult may simply be an innocent comment or observation.

Some experts believe this new awareness and sensitivity serves a purpose in preparing you to understand the needs of an infant who cannot communicate with words. Perhaps by learning to look at things form several angles, you are learning the skills you'll need to decipher the language of your newborn.

PREVENTION

What to Do

❑ Keep your body healthy and fit by doing the following:
- Eat a well-balanced diet, including plenty of fresh fruits and vegetables, whole grains, milk products, and protein-rich foods, such as cheese, fish, chicken, legumes, and meat.

- Exercise several times a week. Try to walk outdoors every day, even if it's just a few blocks during your lunch break.
- Get plenty of R&R—rest and recreation. Go window-shopping, go on a picnic, or make an appointment for a free make-up makeover at a department store beauty counter.

❑ Read about pregnancy and parenting. Read about how it affects your partner and other family members, as well as yourself.

❑ Enroll in early pregnancy classes during the first trimester and childbirth education classes in the second or third trimester. There you and your partner will find professional guidance from your teacher and group support and understanding from other expectant parents.

❑ Talk out your concerns with those nearest you. You're more vulnerable now to criticism , whether real or imagined. You may feel insecure about your ability to meet the demands of pregnancy and birth or to fulfill the role of mother. Let your family and friends know that you'll need their patience for a while.

❑ Realize that your spouse, your parents, and your children, if any, are going through a transition too. They need the same kind of love and support you do. Talk with one another.

❑ Learn to trust yourself. Most women have perfectly healthy pregnancies, resulting in perfectly healthy babies. And most parents just naturally do the right things for their baby.

What to Avoid

❑ Avoid overloading yourself with commitments at work or at home. Pregnancy is a time to conserve your mental and physical energy as much as possible.

❑ Avoid overanalyzing statements, actions, and situations. When you're pregnant, a suggestion can sound like a criticism. For now, it's probably wise to assume that people mean well and are only trying to help. For example, if you find yourself gritting your teeth as your mother tells you that you shouldn't go swimming during pregnancy or as she cautions you for the hundredth time not to stretch your arms above your head while you're pregnant, you can ignore her, yell at her, or explain why this is not dangerous. If you ignore her, she'll probably do it again. If you yell at her, her feelings will be hurt, and you'll feel guilty. But if you thank her for her concern, and then show her a book on prenatal anatomy or exercise, she just might understand and stop offering unsolicited advice.

COMFORT

What to Do

❑ If you find yourself swinging from one mood to another, review the preventive tips above.

❑ If a situation is unavoidable, or if avoidance is a problem, confront it head on. Very few situations improve if you ignore them. It may work with people you'll never meet again, but with family and friends the best thing to do is to confront them. Before you do, answer for yourself the following questions.

1. What is the problem?
2. Whose problem is it?
3. Why does it bother me?
4. What are my alternatives?
5. What are the consequences of each alternative?
6. Which one do I choose?

By working this out ahead of time, you'll know what you want to say and accomplish when you confront the person. When you state the problem, it helps to use "I-language." Instead of saying, "You bother me when you... ," say, "I feel uncomfortable (or hurt, or angry, or sad) when I hear..." This sounds less like an attack. You're simply telling someone how you feel about something.

(*See also* Dreams, page 50; Fatigue, page 53; Insomnia, page 79; and Sexual Adjustments, page 98.)

Multiple Pregnancy

If you're expecting more than one baby, you're probably experiencing the same concerns as other expectant parents, along with the special problems and joys of a multiple pregnancy. About one in every eighty births in America results in twins, which means that one of every forty babies is a twin. Triplets occur only once in every 10,000 births, and quadruplets, quintuplets, and larger sets of multiples are even rarer.

You'll go through the same physical changes in a multiple pregnancy as any other expectant mother. But, because your body is supporting more than one baby, some of the discomforts will be intensified. In her book *Having Twins* (Houghton Mifflin Co., 1980), Elizabeth Noble points out that, by the thirty-second week of a twin pregnancy, the mother's uterus is already the size of a full-term uterus in a singleton pregnancy. This greater, more rapid weight gain often causes increased difficulty with backaches, shortness of breath, and urinary frequency. You'll also be more vulnerable to heartburn, constipation, and swelling, as well as hemorrhoids and varicose veins. And the added burden on your heart, lungs, and kidneys means you'll probably experience more fatigue, too.

Although this list of problems may be discouraging, you can do a great deal to reduce your discomfort by making sure you take proper care of yourself.

PREVENTION

What to Do

❏ Obviously, you can't prevent a multiple pregnancy, but you can prevent some of the difficulties that may accompany it. To prevent a specific discomfort, refer to the Contents page of this book.

❏ Enroll in early pregnancy classes and in a childbirth preparation course. Cesarean birth is more common among mothers of multiples, so talk with your childbirth educator about special classes.

How Are Twins Formed?

Approximately two-thirds of twins are *fraternal*, meaning the babies came from two eggs, each of which was fertilized by a different sperm. They share the same genetic relationship as any brothers or sisters. They may or may not look like one another and may not even be of the same sex. Because they start out as two distinct embryos, each fraternal twin has its own amniotic sac and placenta. This fact is sometimes used at birth to determine whether the twins are fraternal or identical. It's not always possible to tell, though, because the placentas may fuse together during the pregnancy, making them appear as one.

Identical twins come from the joining of a single egg and a single sperm that, shortly after fertilization, splits in two. They share the same features and are the same sex. About 25 percent are "mirror twins," meaning some of their identical features are on opposite sides, so that each child seems to reflect the mirror image of the other. Identical twins usually have separate amniotic sacs, but share a placenta. Sometimes there are two placentas, but only rarely do they share both placenta and amniotic sac.

Triplets can be identical too, with one egg splitting into three separate embryos. But, more often they begin as separate eggs, or as two eggs, one of which splits to form a third embryo. When this happens, two of the babies are identical, and the third is their fraternal triplet. Larger sets of multiples, such as quadruplets and quintuplets, can be formed the same way.

❑ A multiple pregnancy means a higher risk for premature birth. You can give your babies a better chance at a healthy and timely birth by taking good care of yourself.

Here's how:

- Eat a balanced diet that includes plenty of whole grains, milk products, fresh fruits and vegetables, and protein-rich food, such as fish, chicken, beef, cheese, beans and eggs. Keep in mind that you need an extra 300-500 calories a day while expecting twins.
- Drink eight to ten glasses of water a day.
- Get plenty of rest. Bearing twins places an added burden on your body, so it's important that you get enough rest. Here are a few suggestions that can help.

    Arrange for someone else to do the shopping and cooking and household chores. If you can't afford to hire someone, turn to family and friends. The next time someone offers to help, ask them to pick up your dry cleaning or do some grocery shopping for you. If no one offers, ask. And, if all else fails, let some of these jobs go for a while.

    If this is not your first child, you may want to arrange for someone to care for your child each day while you rest.

    If you're employed outside your home, your doctor will probably advise you to take an earlier maternity leave than you had planned.

❑ Discuss with your husband how you'll deal with the many changes your babies may bring. Your feelings about having twins may vary from one day to the next, or even one moment to the next, and you may sometimes find yourself wishing you were expecting only one. After all, if having one baby reduces the amount of time and energy you have for yourself, having two reduces it even further. Twins will also make your house or apartment seem smaller than before, and they may have the same effect on your financial resources. You and your husband will be extra busy after the birth, so it's imperative that you both take time now to talk about it.

❑ Contact the local Mothers of Twins Club. Thousands of parents share the same joys and the same doubts as you. For many of them, a local Mothers of Twins Club has provided the support needed for an easier, more satisfying transition into parenthood. If you're interested in learning more about caring for and living with twins, contact the National Organization of Mothers of Twins Clubs, Inc., at 12404 Princess Jeanne NE, Albuquerque, New Mexico, 87112-4640.

FACT OR FICTION?

"Twins always skip a generation."
"Twins run on the father's side."

Neither of these beliefs is true. Each generation of a particular family has the same chance to bear twins. And, while the father's genetic background has no effect on the rate of multiple conceptions, the mother's does. Your chances are increased if your family history includes twins. If you've already given birth to a set of fraternal twins, your chances of doing it again are quadrupled. Your chances of conceiving twins increases with your age, weight, and height, and are greater with each successive pregnancy.

What to Do

❑ For help with a specific discomfort, refer to the Contents page of this book.

❑ Talk with your birth attendant and your childbirth educator about exercises to help relieve or reduce many of the discomforts you're feeling. You'll probably experience more discomforts than other expectant mothers, so you'll need to pay more attention to preventing or relieving them.

Nasal Congestion

"I know it sounds silly, but I think I might be allergic to pregnancy. I started sniffing before I even knew I was pregnant, and I've been sniffing ever since."

For some women, pregnancy feels like one very long cold, and more than one expectant mother has asked me if it's possible to be allergic to pregnancy. No, you can't be allergic to pregnancy, but you can have a nine-month case of the sniffles. The problem is that the hormonal changes of pregnancy tend to dry out your body's mucous membranes. And, because your nose is lined with mucous membrane, you may end up with *rhinitis*, or swollen, inflamed nasal passage. That's why it sometimes feels like you can't breathe through your nose. Sniffing and blowing your nose probably won't help, but there are a few measures you can take to be more comfortable.

PREVENTION

What to Do

❑ Fill an empty nasal spray bottle or nose dropper with warm water and use it to insert a few drops into your nose several times a day.

❑ If your house or work place has a dry atmosphere, use a humidifier. (Be sure to keep it properly cleaned in order to prevent the growth of mold or fungus that could be released into the air.)

❑ If you don't have a humidifier, you can use the old home remedy of keeping a pot of water boiling on the stove. Just be sure to check it often so the water doesn't boil away and burn the pot.

❑ Fill a pot with water and let it come to a boil. Then, *take it off the burner* and lean your head over the water and inhale the steam. Hold a towel over your head to keep in the steam, and be sure you don't get close enough to the heat to burn the delicate tissue inside your nose.

(If you like, add mint leaves or a teaspoon of oil of eucalyptus to the water.)

What to Avoid

❑ Avoid decongestants and nasal sprays. Even though they're available without a prescription, they're still drugs. They can raise your blood pressure and their safety in pregnancy has not been proven.

COMFORT

What to Do

❑ For nasal or sinus congestion, apply pressure to the indentation between your eyebrows and on either side of the lower, outer edge of each nostril (see figure on this page). Hold pressure on each point for at least one minute. (Or apply a hot, wet washcloth across your nose and eyes.) If your sinuses needed to drain, you should feel it begin within fifteen minutes.
❑ Notify your doctor if you develop symptoms of a sinus infection, such as fever, earache, or pain.

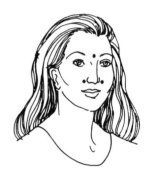

*Pressure Points to Relieve
Nasal Congestion*

What to Avoid

❑ See Prevention tips, "What to Avoid."

Nausea/Vomiting

"I wake up every morning, march into the bathroom, and promptly throw up. Then I go start Dave's breakfast."

"What's the worst thing about pregnancy? I'll tell you—it's waking up every morning to the sound of my wife's throwing up in the bathroom."

Morning sickness is one of the earliest signs of pregnancy for many women. About 70 percent will experience nausea at some time. It usually begins in the first weeks of pregnancy and ends by the fourth month, but for 12 percent this problem will continue for the entire nine months. And it may not be just in the morning. As one woman said, "Morning sickness? How about calling it twenty-four-hour sickness?"

Some experts think there's an emotional cause for morning sickness. Others blame hormonal changes that lead to an increased level of stomach acid. Still others think low blood sugar may be a factor. This temporary condition can occur in pregnancy due to the excessive protein requirements of the developing fetus. If you're not eating well, your blood sugar will be low, and this can cause nausea, headaches, and fatigue. The problem is more pronounced in the morning because it's been so long since you've eaten. At the same time, your empty stomach has been secreting acid, which further nauseates you. There are a number of effective, natural remedies to prevent or relieve morning sickness, no matter what time of day it occurs. But, even if you don't obtain full relief, you can take heart in knowing that recent studies have found nausea during pregnancy to be associated with good fetal health.

PREVENTION

What to Do

❑ Make sure your diet contains sufficient amounts of protein and complex carbohydrates. You need three or four daily servings of high-protein foods, such as fish, chicken, beans, cheese, or meat, and four daily servings of complex carbohydrates, such as whole grains and fresh fruits and vegetables.

❑ At your bedside, keep a piece of chocolate candy or several soda crackers to eat before arising in the morning.

❑ Some nutrition experts also recommend a vitamin B_6 supplement to reduce and prevent nausea. Don't take megadoses: 75-100 milligrams should be enough.

What to Avoid

❑ Avoid greasy or spicy foods.

COMFORT

What to Do

❑ Drink a glass of milk or take two calcium tablets to neutralize the acid.

❑ Suck or chew ice chips.

❑ Eat an apple or potato without the peeling. Many women find this helps reduce the effects of stomach acid.

❑ Apply a cold cloth or ice pack to your throat.

❑ Breathe slowly in and out through your mouth while using any relaxation technique described in this book.

❑ Apply pressure or cold to one or both of the points shown in figure on page 69. These points are located just behind the *mastoid processes,* which lie in back of each ear. To find the points, place your finger just below the lower ridge of bone at the back of your skull. Now, move your finger toward the back of your ear until you feel the bone start to curve downward, just behind the ear. That's it!

❑ Chamomile tea relieves nausea for some women, but others cannot tolerate it when they're nauseated.

❑ *Report persistent vomiting to your physician.*

What to Avoid

❑ Avoid unnecessary emotional or physical stress. Nausea sometimes is aggravated by emotional and physical strain, so don't take on extra responsibilities at home or at work until after your baby is born. Keep in mind that this is not a good time to change houses or jobs, or to entertain large groups of friends or relatives. Allow yourself to take it easy and relax now. (Refer to the section on Moods, page 83, if you think your nausea may be related to emotional strain.)

LABOR TIPS

Nausea is frequently a problem during labor because your digestion slows down. Reducing your food intake when labor starts will decrease your chance of developing nausea. Here's how to relieve any nausea that may occur:

❑ Chew or suck on ice chips.

❑ Suck on peppermint candy.

❑ Apply ice or pressure to the massage points located behind your ears. (See "Comfort, What to Do," above.)

   (*See also* Heartburn, page 74.)

When Daddy Wants Pickles and Ice Cream

About ten to twenty percent of expectant fathers experience pregnancy-related discomforts. Often referred to as the *couvade syndrome*, this male manifestation of pregnancy symptoms may take the form of weight gain, bloating, backaches, cravings, or—you guessed it—morning sickness.

We don't know why this happens to some men. Perhaps it's a man's way of sharing what his partner is going through or of helping her "carry" the baby. One couple from my classes demonstrated this beautifully when they answered the two questions I always use on opening night:

"What's been the best thing about the pregnancy? What's been the worst?" Here's what they said:

She: "The best thing about this pregnancy is that I haven't had any morning sickness."
He: "The worst thing about this pregnancy is that *I've* had all the morning sickness!"

There's no quick cure for male morning sickness, but it should disappear soon after the baby is born. Meanwhile, the comfort measures described in this section should help.

Navel Discomfort

During the last few months of pregnancy you may feel uncomfortable twinges or a pulling sensation in or around your navel, or belly button. You'll probably also notice that it protrudes quite a bit. (Or, as one of my clients put it: "All of a sudden I have an 'outie'!") This central portion of the belly where the muscles of your abdomen meet is usually weaker than the surrounding parts. As your baby grows, your muscles stretch, which can weaken them further. This leaves your navel with less support, which can result in the soreness you feel.

COMFORT

What to Do

❑ Use positions and exercises that take weight off your abdomen or that strengthen your abdominal muscle wall. These include the Kneeling Pelvic Tilt (page 19), the Standing Pelvic Tilt (page 10), and the Buttocks Curl (page 11).

❏ Use Abdominal Effleurage (page 40).

(*See also* Abdominal Pressure, page 4; and Backache, page 15.)

Nosebleeds

You may have noticed that your nasal passages are drier now, due to hormonal changes. These changes also tend to make the blood vessels in the nose more delicate, which means you may experience nose-bleeds.

PREVENTION

What to Do

❏ Increase the humidity in your home (see page 90).
❏ Fill a nasal spray bottle or nose dropper with warm water and insert several drops into your nose at regular intervals throughout the day.
❏ Be sure you get plenty of vitamin C daily. This cell-strengthening nutrient is found in citrus fruit, broccoli, potatoes, onions, and tomatoes.

COMFORT

What to Do

❏ To stop a nosebleed, pinch the nostrils shut for about ten minutes. Be sure to hold it for a full ten minutes, by the clock, before checking for further bleeding. The stimulation of pinching and releasing intermittently in order to check the nose often increases the bleeding. An ice pack applied to the bridge of the nose may also help. If after ten minutes there is still bleeding, try packing the nostril with absorbent cotton or gauze, and then pinch it closed for another ten minutes. If this doesn't help, you may need to call your doctor or an emergency clinic for further help.

(*See also* Nasal Congestion, page 90.)

Pelvic Pressure

The increased flow of blood throughout your body places a strain on all your blood vessels, especially those in the pelvic and vaginal area, and often results in a feeling of pressure and tenderness here. During late pregnancy, the weight of your baby presses on these vessels, adding to the strain and preventing a good return of blood from this region back to your heart. This creates an excess of blood that may make the labia (the lips of the vagina) appear bruised and swollen. Along with this, you may feel a sense of pelvic congestion accompanied by a throbbing soreness. For some women this discomfort is more pronounced during love-making, when sexual arousal further increases the blood flow to these tissues. Some women notice relief after orgasm, but others are still uncomfortable, and may even be reluctant to engage in sexual activity because of this problem.

COMFORT

What to Do

- ❏ When resting, place pillows under your hips. The elevation helps the blood return from the lower body to the heart, making you more comfortable.
- ❏ Use the Knee-Chest position (page 7) and the Bridge (page 7) to reduce excess bloodflow to the area.
- ❏ Use the Kegel exercise (page 28) to help improve the flow of blood into and out of the pelvic area.
- ❏ If you are very uncomfortable, try placing an ice pack on the outside of your vagina to numb the tissue and at the same time reduce the amount of blood in the area.

What to Avoid

- ❏ Do not apply heat to the vaginal area — it will encourage more blood to flow to the pelvis, and may aggravate your problem.

 ## LABOR TIPS

Pelvic pressure is often quite strong during late labor. For relief, try these massage techniques:

- ❏ Apply pressure to either side of your spine, just above your tailbone (just above where your buttocks join). Your partner can do this for you, or you can do it by lying on your fists.

❏ Apply pressure on both sides of your pelvis, where the hipbone juts out to the front. Place your thumbs here, as though you were trying to hook them under the bone, and press.

(*See also* Hemorrhoids, page 75; and Vaginal Varicose Veins, page 113.)

Rib Discomfort

Each time you breathe, your rib cage expands and contracts to help you move air in and out. In the last half of pregnancy, your growing baby pushes your abdominal organs up toward your chest, forcing your rib cage to remain more expanded than usual. This constant tension in the muscles and ligaments in your chest wall may leave your ribs and upper back feeling weary and sore.

COMFORT

What to Do

❏ Use Super-Dooper Arm Reaches (page 60), the Standing Complete Breath (page 35), and the Sitting Deep Breath (page 34) to help relieve some of the tension and discomfort of aching rib muscles.

❏ Use the Chest Expander (this page) if your problem seems to be mostly your upper back. Also, try the exercises and massage techniques suggested for upper backache on page 17.

❏ Use The Balloon relaxation technique (page 163). When doing The Balloon for rib discomfort, move the imaginary balloon from your abdomen to your lungs. As you inhale and feel the balloon inflate, you'll notice a cool breath of energy enter your lungs. As you exhale and feel the balloon deflate, you'll feel warmth and relaxation as the balloon seems to go limp and your chest muscles let go.

EXERCISE TECHNIQUES

CHEST EXPANDER

Benefits: Eases upper backache, eases rib fatigue and soreness, and eases shortness of breath.

1. Stand with your feet about twelve to eighteen inches apart and clasp your hands together behind your back.
2. Inhale, lifting your arms up behind you as far as you can. (To lift your arms higher, keep your hands clasped and turn them outward.)
3. Place one foot forward and exhale as you bend to the front.
4. Hold this position for a count of three.
5. Inhale and slowly return to an erect position.
6. Exhale and slowly drop your arms.

(*See also* Backache, page 15; and Breathlessness, page 33.)

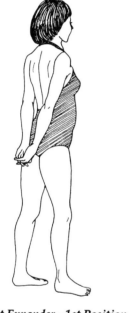

Chest Expander—1st Position

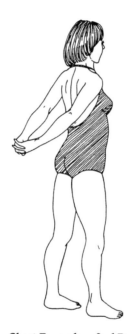

Chest Expander—2nd Position

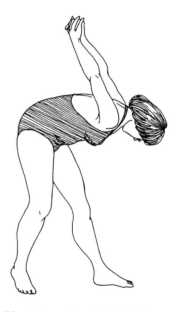

Chest Expander—3rd Position

Sexual Adjustments

A quick look at the list of pregnancy-related discomforts noted on the Contents page provides a clue to why your sex life may not be the same as it was before you conceived. Abdominal pressure and shortness of breath can make intercourse uncomfortable and chronic fatigue can leave you with little energy or desire for sexual activities. Backache and weight gain can make it difficult to find a comfortable position, and concerns about urinary frequency may inhibit or distract you. Other changes that can contribute to a decline in your interest in sex include breast tenderness, excessive fetal activity, gas, pelvic pressure, and nausea.

You can reduce many of the physical discomforts that hinder your enjoyment of sex by following the comfort measures given in this book for each complaint. But you may experience other problems more directly related to your sexual activities. For example, you may find that your usual positions for intercourse just don't work now. Deep penetration may be uncomfortable and lying on your back may make it difficult to breathe.

Besides the physical barriers, you or your partner may also be worried about your baby's safety, a concern that may be reinforced by the increased fetal and uterine activity that often accompanies or follows intercourse. If yours is a healthy pregnancy, there's no need for concern. It's normal for the baby, who is floating in fluid, to feel a bit jostled by the movements you and your partner are making, and to respond by waking up and moving himself. He doesn't know what you're doing; he only knows that someone is rocking his boat. His movements may be attempts to get you to settle down so he can go back to sleep, or he may be showing his enjoyment of the rocking motion. Even the uterine contractions that follow orgasm are normal. These are usually Braxton-Hicks, or practice contractions, that won't cause labor to start unless it's just about time for the baby to be born, or if you've had bouts with premature labor.

Sometimes the sex drive changes you experience are due to emotional factors. You may be worried that you don't look as appealing as you did before the pregnancy. Your husband may have negative feelings about making love with a pregnant woman. He may in some way feel threatened by your pregnancy. If, like most women, your conversation is devoted mostly to the baby, the pregnancy, what the doctor said, and the latest book you read on the subject, he may fear that you care more about the baby than about him. Both of you may have concerns about how your lives or relationships are changing. These all are factors in determining your feelings about sex and sexuality.

Although we've been discussing how pregnancy can decrease your sex drive, it is important to point out that for many people the opposite is true. Some women feel more feminine than ever and some men feel they've proven their masculinity. This can be a powerful aphrodisiac for either person. Most couples find that their desire for sex fluctuates throughout the pregnancy.

PREVENTION

What to Do

☐ Try new positions for lovemaking. Right now, the classic position of the man on top and the woman on the bottom may be uncomfortable. You may feel more relaxed lying side by side facing each other, or with the woman on top so that she has a little more control over the depth of penetration. It may take a while to find the most comfortable positions, but if you look at it as an interesting challenge, you just might have fun!

☐ Talk with one another. Tell your partner what you want, what you like, what you don't like. Ask him to show you what he wants, too. Often it's not just the fears and concerns that hamper a healthy relationship, but also the lack of communication between partners. If you talk with each other about these matters, you can better understand what is happening. Silence only magnifies the problems.

☐ Consider other ways to express your physical love for each other. Intercourse is not the only way to say, "I love you." Cuddling and petting convey love and affection and, for many women, can be as satisfying as intercourse.

☐ Use the Total Back Massage (page 23) and other massage techniques described throughout this book to share your affection for one another and to help you relax together.

☐ Make a pact with your partner to work together to achieve a new closeness that will fortify your relationship now and through the difficult period of new parenthood.

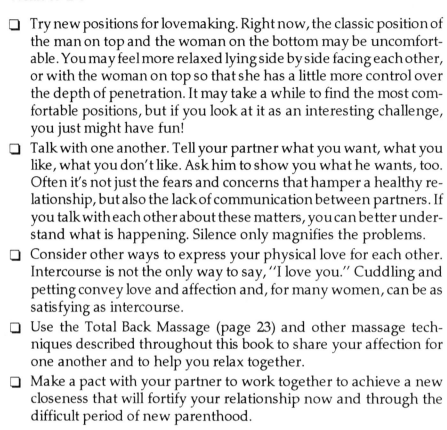

When Should You Avoid Sexual Intercourse?

Experts disagree about wisdom of continuing sexual intercourse during certain times of the pregnancy. The most common and commonsense advice is that, if you have a healthy pregnancy, intercourse is usually safe until the mucous plug has fallen out of the cervix or the bag of waters has begun to leak. Some doctors also advise that you abstain in the first three months at the time you normally would expect your period. This would be during the second, sixth, and tenth weeks, when some women seem more vulnerable to miscarriage. If you've had a previous preterm birth, if this pregnancy has been threatened by bouts with preterm labor, or if you have had any cramping or bleeding, you should consult your obstetrician before engaging in any form of lovemaking that might cause orgasm.

What to Avoid

❑ Don't keep your fears and concerns about your sexual life to yourself. Share them with your partner. Open communication will lessen the chances of the problems becoming magnified.

COMFORT

What to Do

❑ See Prevention tips.

(*See also* Mood Changes, page 83; and refer to the other sections according to your specific needs.)

Skin Changes

Pregnancy affects almost every part of your body, including your skin. While most of these changes aren't uncomfortable, they can be annoying.

Blemishes

Pregnancy works wonders for the complexions of some women, clearing up pimples and reducing blackheads. But for others, even those who have never had a complexion problem, the opposite is true. (In high school I always felt left out because I was the only teenager I knew who had never developed a pimple. In fact, I didn't have a single blemish until my first pregnancy, when I was twenty-one.) Pregnancy can cause blemishes because the hormonal changes make your sweat glands and sebaceous, or oil-producing, glands work overtime.

PREVENTION

What to Do

❑ Keep your facial skin clean and free of excess oil.

❏ If your complexion is particularly oily, try this routine:

- Use a rough washcloth or cleansing granules on your face once a week.
- Follow this with a clay-based facial mask or an astringent to temporarily shrink pores.
- Each day, use a pH-balanced cleansing bar with warm water, followed by a mild astringent—either a commercial solution or the juice of a lemon—to tighten the pores.
- If you use a moisturizer, apply it only to the dry areas of your face, such as your cheeks and around your eyes.

What to Avoid

❏ Avoid overworking your facial skin by too vigorous or too frequent cleaning.

❏ Avoid oil-based make-ups.

❏ Avoid applying too much moisturizer.

COMFORT

What to Do

❏ If a pimple has a definite head, cleanse the area with alcohol and use a sharp, sterile needle to pierce the edge of the pustule, gently expressing the contents. Follow this with a dab of alcohol.

❏ Consult your obstetrician before using medicated skin creams.

What to Avoid

❏ Avoid squeezing pimples. This could force the bacteria to go deeper and the infection might enter your bloodstream, affecting you and the baby.

❏ *Avoid using the medication Accutane.* It can cause serious birth defects in your baby.

Color Changes

Pregnancy hormones affect your skin's color by causing extra *melanin*, the substance responsible for freckles and suntans, to be deposited in certain areas of your body. As a result, your nipples darken and a line called the *linea negra* develops from the umbilicus down to the pubic area. These and other color changes are usually more pronounced in brunettes than in women with lighter hair and skin. After your baby is born, the linea negra will probably disappear, and while your nipples will never return to their former shade, their color should lighten. Perhaps the most annoying skin change for many women is the appearance of dark patches across the forehead, cheeks, and nose. Called *chloasma,* or "mask of pregnancy," this darkening is intensified by sunlight or tanning lamps. (This continues to be true for many women years after the pregnancy is over.) Chloasma almost always fades after the baby is born, but it may not disappear.

Some expectant mothers complain that their complexion becomes sallow in early pregnancy, and then turns ruddy close to birth. As with chloasma, this change usually disappears or becomes less noticeable after the birth.

COMFORT

(As with many changes of pregnancy, skin discolorations are caused by hormonal changes and cannot be prevented. They can, however, be minimized.)

What to Do

❑ If you spend much time outdoors, ask your doctor about using a sunscreen to help reduce the sun's darkening effect on your facial skin.

❑ Minimize the appearance of facial discolorations with a liquid foundation and cover cream in the shade closest to your natural color. If this doesn't help, apply a green undercover cream before the foundation to help even out your skin tone.

❑ Treat yourself to one of the free facials and makeup consultations offered by many beauty salons and department stores. If you enjoy wearing makeup or if you've always wanted to give it a try, this is a good opportunity to learn some new tricks and to ask the experts for free professional guidance in choosing and using makeup.

What to Avoid

❑ Avoid sunlight unless your face is protected with sunscreen.

❑ Avoid trying to get a suntan, either from sunlamps or the real thing, unless you're willing to accept what might be a lifetime of facial blotching and, even more important, of risk for skin cancer.

Rashes

Some pregnant women develop rashes that may or may not be associated with pregnancy. The most common is *miliaria,* or prickly heat, which results from a combination of dampness, friction, and heat. An irritating, red rash, prickly heat is most likely to develop where one part of your body rubs against another over a prolonged time. For example, if your baby's weight makes your lower abdomen sag until it rubs against your pubic area, you'll probably have a problem with prickly heat. It may also occur just beneath your breasts or on your inner thighs.

PREVENTION

What to Do

- ❑ To treat or prevent prickly heat, bathe frequently, then pat the area dry and apply unscented talcum powder.
- ❑ Consult your birth attendant if you develop a rash and are unsure of the cause, or if the rash is preceded or accompanied by fever or the symptoms of a cold.

What to Avoid

- ❑ Avoid tight or restrictive clothing.
- ❑ Avoid panty hose in hot or humid weather.
- ❑ Avoid clothing made of tightly woven cloth or other material that does not allow for evaporation. Examples are leather, vinyl, taffeta, satin, nylon, and finished silk.

COMFORT

What to Do

- ❑ See Prevention tips, "What to Do," above.
- ❑ To ease the irritation, you may find it helpful to apply a cream recommended for diaper rash. If cream doesn't help or if the rash worsens, discontinue its use. Be aware that rashes usually heal faster when exposed to air.

❏ A bath in warm water with baking soda may soothe itching.

❏ A bath in cold water can relieve itching for several hours.

❏ An ice pack applied to a particularly itchy area may offer temporary relief.

What to Avoid

❏ See Prevention tips, "What to Avoid," above.

Spider Veins

You may have noticed tiny broken blood vessels under the surface of your skin. Called *spider nevi* or *spider veins*, they resemble a tiny red spider web. They're more common in pregnancy because of the increased amount of fluid in your bloodstream, but they can also result from high blood pressure, excessive alcohol intake, exposure to high temperatures, or any situation that places added pressure on the blood vessels.

Spider veins aren't painful, but they can be annoying because of their appearance. They occur most frequently on the legs, but some women develop spider veins on the face during delivery because they push so hard that they literally break tiny facial blood vessels.

PREVENTION

What to Avoid

❏ Avoid alcoholic beverages.

❏ Avoid exposure to excessive heat.

❏ Avoid lifting heavy objects.

❏ Avoid prolonged standing.

COMFORT

What to Do

❏ Camouflage the veins with one of the cover creams now available for disguising small scars or birthmarks.

❏ If creams aren't effective and if you find the broken veins particularly annoying or unattractive, a physician can treat them by injecting them with chemicals. (This should wait until after your baby is born.) More than one treatment may be required, and the spider veins may recur.

(*See also* Stretch Marks, below.)

Stress

See Headaches; Insomnia; Mood Changes.

Stretch Marks

The most common cosmetic question I'm asked is, "How can I prevent stretch marks?" These purplish or pink streaks are called *striae gravidarum,* which is Latin for "stripes of pregnancy." They usually appear on the lower abdomen, breasts, thighs, and buttocks, and tend to radiate outward from the center of the body, or to run in parallel or converging patterns. Their distribution follows the pattern of your own weight gain in pregnancy.

Stretch marks, or striae, result from the breakdown of tissue in the deeper, less elastic layers of your skin. There's some evidence to suggest that striae may be related to hormonal changes, but it's more likely that they're caused by just what their name indicates — stretching. You have a greater chance of developing stretch marks if this is your first pregnancy, or if you're a blonde or are overweight. You may not notice any marks during pregnancy, but later, when the over-stretched skin is looser, they may show up. They'll slowly fade to a pearly white or silver color, but they'll never disappear completely.

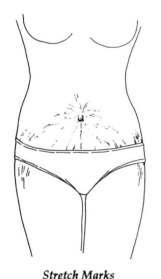

Stretch Marks

PREVENTION

What to Do

❑ Exercise regularly, focusing on the abdomen, hips, and thighs, which are the areas most prone to stretch marks. This will help strengthen the muscles that support your skin and may prevent some of the natural breakdown that occurs during pregnancy.

- For the abdomen, try the Kneeling Pelvic Tilt (see page 19), the Standing Pelvic Tilt (see page 10), or the Buttocks Curl (see page 11).
- For hips and thighs, try walking, swimming, or stationary bicycling. Also try Leg Stretches (see page 45) or Wall Push-Ups (see page 46).
- For the breast, you can strengthen and tone the chest muscles underneath, although you can't actually exercise the breast (since it is not a muscle). Try Wall Push-Ups (see page 46), Chest Expander (see page 97), or Chest Press (below) to improve support to the breasts and help reduce the possibility of stretch marks.

❏ Wear a well-fitting, supportive bra. This will reduce your risk of stretch marks due to the effects of gravity on your breasts as they increase in weight.

What to Avoid

❏ Avoid restricting your weight gain. This will not prevent stretch marks and can hurt both you and your baby.

COMFORT

What to Do

❏ Use a camouflage cream if you're bothered by exposed stretch marks.
❏ Use a non-perfumed cream or lotion to reduce the dryness and itching associated with over-stretched skin.

What to Avoid

❏ Avoid wasting money on expensive creams and lotions that are supposed to prevent or minimize stretch marks. They may reduce dryness and itching, but they cannot prevent stretch marks.

EXERCISE TECHNIQUES

CHEST PRESS

Benefits: Tones chest wall muscles to help support breast tissue.

1. Place your palms together in front of you and inhale.

2. Press your palms against each other while exhaling to a slow count of three.
3. Release and inhale.
4. Repeat five times.

Comments: Be sure to exhale as you press. This is important to help prevent circulatory difficulties during the exercise.

Swelling

By the eighth month of pregnancy you'll probably have experienced some fluid retention and swelling. This is a normal and healthy response. Even women who show no obvious signs of swelling carry about fifteen extra pounds of liquid in their bodies during pregnancy. But, even though a certain amount fluid retention is necessary, too much can be uncomfortable and may result in high blood pressure and other problems.

Each woman retains fluid according to her individual needs. An overweight woman will add more liquid weight during pregnancy, and a thin woman will add more fat. Fluid retention increases in pregnancy for a number of reasons. For example, hormonal changes cause fluid to be retained in the spaces between the body's cells. This is why your face seems rounder and your features softer. Fluid retention also helps you produce a continual supply of amniotic fluid for your baby. This liquid, which fills the bag of waters, protects your baby from bumps and jolts and temperature changes. Your baby also drinks the liquid and urinates into it. Your body has to filter and replace the amniotic fluid on a contin-uous basis, and this requires a ready supply of fluid in your own body.

The fluid volume in your bloodstream increases by about 42 percent by the thirty-fourth week. You need a greater volume of circulating blood to help meet the demands of nourishing your baby and getting rid of waste products. This extra blood volume slows down your circulation and that, along with the extra fluid in the body's tissues, is what causes swelling, or *edema.*

In late pregnancy the pressure of your growing baby, combined with the increased blood volume, makes it even more difficult for blood to return from your arms and legs to your heart. The problem is greatest in your legs, where both gravity and the weight of your uterus on the veins slow down the return flow. This is why the most common sites for swelling are the ankles and feet.

How Much Swelling Is Too Much?

Health professionals usually refer to two kinds of swelling, or edema. *Dependent edema* is caused by the position of the affected body part. When you sit or stand for a long time, your feet are in a dependent position; that is, they're lower than the rest of your body. As a result, gravity works against your veins as they attempt to move the blood from your legs back up to your heart. The swelling that results is temporary. If you elevate your legs for a few minutes, it will disappear.

Pitting edema is more serious because it usually indicates that your body is retaining too much fluid. It's identified by puffiness, especially in the face, around the eyes, or in the hands. Unlike dependent edema, this type of swelling doesn't disappear when you elevate the affected part. One way to tell the difference between puffiness and normal swelling is to do the "cake test." If you indent the top of a freshly baked cake with your finger and it doesn't spring back, the cake isn't quite done. Try the same test on yourself. If you indent the swollen area on your ankles or feet and, instead of springing back quickly, it leaves a dent, that area is puffy, or too swollen. (The term "pitting edema" refers to this temporary dent, or pit, left in your skin.")

Report to your doctor or midwife any sudden increase in swelling, as well as any puffiness in your face, around your eyes, or in your hands. Report pitting edema that occurs anywhere in your body. These changes may signal the onset of *toxemia,* or *pre-eclampsia,* a pregnancy-related condition in which the blood pressure is abnormally high. If your hands are swollen or numb when you first wake up, do the Arm Reaches on page 60. If you slept on your arm and this is causing the swelling, the exercises will reestablish the circulation and will reduce the edema. If they don't help, notify your doctor.

COMFORT

(Swelling is a normal part of pregnancy. The following suggestions will make you more comfortable and can help prevent excessive swelling, which is not a normal part of pregnancy.)

What to Do

❑ Elevate your legs and hips on pillows several times a day and rest in this position for about fifteen or twenty minutes to let gravity work for you.

❑ When sleeping or resting, lie on your left side. This is the best position to take the weight of the uterus off the vena cava, the large blood vessel that returns blood from the legs to the heart. Your left side is best but lying on your right side can help, too.

❑ Walk, swim, or ride a stationary bike four or five times a week to stimulate circulation and help move blood from your legs to your heart.

❏ Sit in a rocking chair when reading, knitting, watching television, etc. As you rock, the muscles in your feet, ankles, and legs contract and relax, helping to squeeze blood back up toward your heart.

❏ Drink at least eight glasses of liquid daily. You need this much to help your kidneys and bladder work efficiently.

❏ Eliminate excess salt from your diet. Besides eliminating the more obvious sources of salt, such as salted nuts and chips, look for hidden sources of salt, such as preserved meats, pickles, and soft drinks. *Do not put yourself on a low-salt diet.* With the extra fluid your system is handling, you need salt, but many Americans eat far too much. Just use enough to flavor your food, and avoid any excess salt.

What to Avoid

❏ *Avoid sleeping or resting on your back after the fourth month.* This places the entire weight of the uterus and baby directly on the vena cava, hampering the bloodflow.

❏ *Do not reduce the amount of fluid you drink.*

❏ *Avoid a low-salt diet.*

❏ *Avoid taking diuretics (water pills).*

(*See also* Weight Gain, page 115.)

Tension

See Headaches; Insomnia; Mood Changes.

Vaginal Discharge

Since early in your pregnancy, you may have noticed a thin, mucous discharge that's pale yellow or almost colorless. This is normal and is just another result of the increased hormonal activity going on inside you.

Look Out for These Discharges

Bleeding. Some women notice light spotting during the first three months of pregnancy at the time when their period would normally occur. This is usually not a problem, but you should report it to your birth attendant, just to be sure. Any other type of vaginal bleeding is *not* normal unless you're within two or three weeks of your due date. By then your cervix will have started to soften and open in preparation for labor, and the mucous plug that had closed it off may fall out. When it does, you may see an actual plug of mucous or you may simply notice a increase in the discharge you were already experiencing. Either way, the mucous will be tinged with blood.

Infection. The constant moisture within your vagina encourages growth of bacteria and viruses. Certain sexually-transmitted diseases can harm you and your baby. In most cases, these infections can be treated with oral or injectable medication or with medicated vaginal suppositories, but it's important to seek help right away in order to prevent complications for you or your baby.

Notify your birth attendant if you notice any of the following signs:

❑ Thickened discharge.
❑ Vaginal burning or itching.
❑ Foul-smelling discharge.
❑ Discharge that is bloody, or any color other than pale yellow or colorless.
❑ Thin, watery discharge that gushes or drips continuously. (Your bag of waters may have broken.)

COMFORT

What to Do

❑ Wear panties with a cotton crotch to allow excess moisture to evaporate.
❑ Use a sanitary pad or panty liner, if necessary.

What to Avoid

❑ Do not douche unless your doctor or midwife recommends it.
❑ Avoid feminine hygiene sprays. They sometimes irritate the delicate tissue of your vagina.
❑ Do not use tampons while you're pregnant. If you feel the need for protection, use a sanitary napkin or panty shield.
❑ Avoid wearing panty hose or other restrictive clothing for more than a couple of hours, if at all.

(*See also* Bladder Infection, page 29.)

Varicose Veins

Varicose Veins, Legs

"How can I prevent varicose veins?" is one of the most common questions I heard when teaching prenatal exercise classes. Most of the moms wanted to know how to avoid varicosities or how to get rid of them. A varicose vein occurs when blood has difficulty flowing out of an area of your body, such as your legs or rectum, and back to the heart. Ordinarily the valves within the blood vessels open and close to force blood back to the heart. But if a valve is weak, the blood may back up inside the vein. This increases the pressure within the vein, which is why varicose veins bulge.

Weak valves seem to run in families. If one or both of your parents has varicose veins, you may have inherited the tendency for weak valves. Whether or not varicosities run in your family, you have a greater risk for developing them just because you're pregnant. The added weight of pregnancy, combined with the increased volume of fluid in your bloodstream forces your valves to work harder to keep the blood flowing smoothly.

Varicose veins aren't always noticeable or uncomfortable. But they can become enlarged and can cause aching and heaviness in the affected area. The most common locations for varicose veins are in the legs and the rectum. (When they happen in the rectum, they're called hemorrhoids. See page 75 for more information.)

PREVENTION

What to Do

❑ Elevate your legs several times a day to encourage blood to flow out of your legs and back to your heart. Lying on your back may impair circulation, so try to get comfortable on your left side with your feet elevated on several pillows. This is the best position for encouraging circulation, but if it doesn't feel good, try your right side. Take your time getting up. Otherwise, the change in bloodflow may cause a temporary drop in blood pressure, making you feel dizzy and unsteady for a few moments.

❑ If you spend a lot of time sitting, use a rocking chair or keep a stool or box under your desk or chair so you can elevate your feet at intervals.

❏ Move about frequently. If you work at a desk, take a few minutes every hour to get up and walk about the room. At lunch save an extra ten minutes for a brisk outdoor walk. When sitting for long periods, life one leg at a time and do ankle circles, first to the right and then to the left. When standing, keep your legs moving, shifting your weight from one to another. Just wiggling your toes will help.

❏ Exercise regularly to improve circulation. Good choices are walking, swimming, and stationary bicycling.

COMFORT

What to Do

❏ See Prevention tips above.

❏ Wear support hose. Maternity support hose are available at maternity shops and pharmacies. Elevate your legs for several minutes before putting on the hose.

❏ Take warm baths to soothe aching legs.

❏ *Notify your birth attendant if you notice an area on your leg that is painful, tender, red, hot, or swollen.* This may be an inflamed vein in which a clot has developed. This is not a condition you should attempt to treat by yourself.

❏ If you have varicose veins that are extremely uncomfortable or if their appearance bothers you a great deal, you may want to talk to your doctor about recommending a surgeon to treat them after your pregnancy.

What to Avoid

❏ *Do not apply deep, kneading massage to your legs while you're pregnant.* Varicose veins increase your risk of developing blood clots, and if you should have any, a vigorous massage could break them loose and let them flow dangerously into the bloodstream.

(*See also* Hemorrhoids, page 75, and Vaginal Varicose Veins, below.)

Varicose Veins, Vaginal

The pressure of your baby and uterus weighs heavily on your pelvic floor, and for some women this results in vaginal varicose veins. These develop the same way as varicosities in the legs and they can be very uncomfortable. Vaginal varicosities are usually less noticeable after your baby is born, but you may be bothered by them at intervals throughout your life, especially if you become pregnant again or gain excessive weight.

COMFORT

What to Do

❑ Use the Knee-Chest exercise (page 7), the Bridge (page 7), and the Kegel exercise (page 28) to help blood flow out of your vaginal area.

❑ Apply an ice pack to your vagina.

What to Avoid

❑ Avoid applying heat to the vaginal area. It probably won't help and may aggravate the problem by drawing more blood to the area.

(*See also* Hemorrhoids, page 75; Pelvic Pressure, page 96; and Varicose Veins, Legs, page 112.)

Visual Disturbances

Visual disturbances, such as double vision or seeing spots or lights, may be symptoms of preeclampsia, or toxemia, and should be reported to your birth attendant. If this is not the cause, the changes may be due to your pregnancy itself. Many women who wear glasses complain that they don't see as well during pregnancy and they wonder if they need a new prescription. The most common complaint of this sort is blurred vision, accompanied by headaches. Perhaps the increased fluid volume of pregnancy changes the pressure in or around the eyes and this temporarily changes the shape of the lens. Whatever the cause, there's little you can do but wait. Even though it may feel like you need new glasses, it doesn't make sense to buy a new pair, because the problem will probably disappear after your baby is born and your body returns to its nonpregnant state.

COMFORT

What to Do

❑ Let your birth attendant know about any headaches or visual disturbances. Consult an ophthalmologist if the blurred vision has become a problem for you.

(*See also* Headaches, page 65.)

Weight Gain

"The worst thing is having to listen to my wife complain about how fat she is. I really hate it when she heads for the bathroom scale, because I know she'll come away depressed."

Extra weight is one of the first pregnancy symptoms to arrive and one of the last to leave. It can be depressing to see yourself getting bigger and bigger, but pregnancy is a package deal—if you want a baby, you have to take the extra weight that goes along with it, at least for now. You should try to gain at least twenty-five to thirty-five pounds before your baby is born. If this seems like a lot, just remember that maternal nutrition and weight gain go hand in hand with good birthweight and strong, healthy babies. If you started pregnancy with some excess weight, or if you're not very active, you won't need to gain as much as a woman who started out underweight or who is very active.

While experts recommend a steady, gradual gain, you may not see any set pattern to how you put on weight. Some women add most of their weight in the first months, while others actually lose weight due to vomiting and nausea. And sometimes the weight seems to come all at once, toward the final months.

Where Do All Those Pounds Go?

The average mother puts on approximately 25 to 35 pounds during pregnancy. These pounds are distributed to the following places. These numbers are averages. No one knows exactly how much weight a particular individual will gain in any of these areas.

6 - 8	Baby	3 - 4	Increased blood volume
2	Uterus	1 - 2	Increased breast size
1.5	Placenta	4	Increased fluid retention
2	Amniotic fluid	4 or more	Stored fat

Quality, Not Quantity

You need about 2,000 to 3,000 calories daily, depending on your weight and activity level. Far more important than the number of calories and pounds, is the quality of food from which they come, so be sure your diet includes plenty of fresh fruits and vegetables, whole grains, milk products, and protein-rich foods, such as fish, chicken, beans, cheese, and meat.

Here's how to make sure that the food you consume is the best for you and your baby:

❑ Avoid foods high in fats, salt, or sugar. (Salt may be listed as sodium and sugar may be listed as sucrose, fructose, dextrose, glucose, corn syrup, or honey.)

❑ When shopping, take time to read labels. Remember, the ingredients are listed in descending order of their quantity in the product. If you don't have time to read labels on each shopping trip, set aside an extra half hour once a month for this.

❑ If you rely on vending machines at work, notice what is available. Many machines carry peanuts and crackers with cheese or peanut butter. Some sell juices and milk. Others offer sandwiches, fruit, and single-serving sizes of canned soups. If you work in a building where the machines are not this versatile, ask the management if they could make some changes. Other employees will welcome nutritious snacks instead of the usual candy bars and soft drinks.

❑ Take-home food can be nutritious if you choose wisely. Unfortunately, it's often very high in sodium and fat. When ordering a hamburger, ask for a single patty with lettuce and tomatoes or onions, as well as cheese (or a milk shake, providing it's made with real milk). This will supply something from every food group. Pizza is a well-balanced meal when topped with meat and cheese, green peppers or onions, and tomato sauce. (For less fat and salt, leave off the meat.) Tacos offer unlimited potential for creative nutrition. (As my mother-in-law said, "A taco is anything with a tortilla wrapped around it." Of course, she said it in Spanish!)

❑ When you buy celery, carrots, mushrooms, and cauliflower, wash and slice them and keep them handy for quick snacks. Raw fruits are satisfying for the sweet tooth and provide a good source of energy and vitamins.

COMFORT

What to Do

❑ For discomforts that may be associated with weight gain, such as backache, fatigue, shortness of breath, and swelling, refer to the Contents page of this book.

❑ Exercise regularly to reduce the uncomfortable effects of weight gain. Walking and stationary bicycling are good choices, but swimming is even better because being in the water reduces your weight by 90 percent . . . until you get out, of course.

❑ Join a prenatal exercise class. Remember, too, that the exercises listed in this book will also help.

(*See also* Cravings, page 47; and Weight, postpartal, page 167.)

Part Two

POSTPARTUM

POSTPARTUM WARNING SIGNS

With all the changes occurring in your body after child-birth, you may have difficulty knowing if something you experience is a natural part of the postpartum period or a sign of a problem. This chart describes the discomforts and danger signs that are most often confused and how to tell the difference. Because no two women are alike, your health-care provider's advice may differ from these suggestions. Please discuss with your birth attendant and your childbirth educator any theraputic measures you take or any questions you have.

PROBLEM	ACTION	CAUSE
BREAST PAIN Nipples are sore or cracked.	Gently massage own milk into nipples. Avoid alcohol, soap, and perfumed creams. If problem persists, contact childbirth educator, midwife, or lactation consultant.	During nursing, nipple probably not centered over baby's tongue or far enough inside her mouth. Baby may be chewing or pulling nipple.
Small, red, tender lump develops on breast.	Nurse more often and longer. Change baby's position during feedings. Hand express remaining milk from breast.	Clogged milk duct.
Breast feels hard, tight, and tender two to five days after birth.	Nurse more often or hand express excess milk. Apply ice packs. (If not nursing, avoid expressing milk. May use acetaminophen for pain.)	Breasts engorged as milk supply comes in.
Tender, reddened area or entire breast is hot and hard. (May also have fever, chills, nausea, or aching.)	NOTIFY YOUR BIRTH ATTENDANT.	May have mastitis (breast infection).
LEG PAIN Painful area is hot, swollen, and red.	NOTIFY YOUR BIRTH ATTENDANT.	May have thrombophlebitis (blood clot with inflammation).
Sharp cramp in calf (charley horse).	Sit with leg straight, foot flexed. Gently stretch upper body toward foot till pain eases.	Cause not definite; may be due to too much or too little calcium.
URINARY DIFFICULTY Urine is dark and concentrated; may have strong odor.	Drink more fluids (at least eight cups of water daily). If problem persists more than 24 hours, *notify birth attendant.*	Insufficient fluid intake.
Urge to urinate is frequent, but little urine is passed and is accompanied by pain. (May have pain in back, side, or lower abdomen. Urine may be dark and concentrated.)	NOTIFY YOUR BIRTH ATTENDANT.	May have cystitis (bladder infection).
VAGINAL DISCHARGE Discharge is rusty or cream colored.	Use sanitary pads. *Do not use tampons.*	Normal postpartum discharge (lochia).
Lochia returns to bright red color.	NOTIFY YOUR BIRTH ATTENDANT.	A piece of placenta may remain inside uterus.
Discharge with pain, itching, foul odor, or foamy texture	NOTIFY YOUR BIRTH ATTENDANT.	May have uterine or vaginal infection.

OTHER WARNING SIGNS
Fever over 100.4° F for more than 24 hours.
Intense, persistent episiotomy pain.
Intense vaginal or pelvic pain.
NOTIFY YOUR BIRTH ATTENDANT.

Many of the comfort measures for postpartum problems are the same as those for similar prenatal problems. After reading the suggestions in this section, look up the corresponding prenatal topic, where you may find more information to help you cope with your discomfort. Whether you had a vaginal or cesarean birth, turn to the specific problem you're experiencing. For example, you'll find comfort measures for the pain of an episiotomy, a laceration, or an abdominal incision listed under "Stitches."

Abdominal Weakness

"I remember lying in bed and looking down at my nice, flat tummy. It was wonderful! But then, I stood up and everything just sort of flopped forward. I looked like I was five months pregnant, except now it was all loose and flabby."

When you were pregnant, you probably looked forward to the time when you could again wear your favorite dresses and tight pants, and when you could look down and see your toes. Eventually that will happen, but right now you're probably disappointed by how your profile looks. After nine months of stretching to make way for your growing baby, it's only natural that the skin and muscles over your abdomen have lost some of their elasticity.

COMFORT

What to Do

❑ Use these exercises to strengthen your abdominal muscle wall:

- Leg Slides (page 122).
- Head Lift (page 123).
- Shoulder Lift (page 123).
- Abdominal Roll (page 124).
- Kneeling Pelvic-Tilt (page 19).
- Standing Pelvic-Tilt (page 10).
- Curl-Ups (page 12).
- Buttocks Curl (page 11).

Your abdominal muscle wall was created to serve as a natural girdle for the mid-section of your body. It will take a while, but with time and a

Checking for Abdominal Muscle Strength

Before doing postpartum exercises, take a few minutes to determine the strength of your abdominal muscles. Here's how:

1. Lie on your back with your knees bent and arms to your sides.

2. As you exhale, slowly lift your head and shoulders about eight inches, keeping your arms out in front of you.

3. With your head and shoulders still elevated, place one hand in the center of your abdomen, just below the navel and press as deeply as you comfortably can. If you feel a soft depression or gap between the two tight bands of muscle on either side of your hand, it means your muscles have separated a bit.

   If you can place only one or two fingers into the width of this gap, you probably have the normal amount of relaxation of muscles and tissues that occurs after giving birth. If the area is wide enough for you to insert more than two fingers, you may have a true separation, or *diastasis recti*. If, after doing this muscle check, you still aren't sure whether you have a separation, repeat the process. This time, begin with your fingers already pressed into the center of your abdomen, just below the navel, before you lift your head and shoulders. This may help you feel the bands of recti muscles move toward the midline as they tighten.

   If you have a diastasis, avoid exercises that involve double leg-lifts and full sit-ups. As you work to tone the muscles, check your progress by periodically measuring how many fingers fit into the gap between the muscles. The gap will narrow as you progress. When you can barely fit even one finger into the space, you'll know that your muscles are strong again.

   (If you experience a severe diastasis recti during pregnancy or delivery, your doctor will want to check it out for you. If exercise and time don't correct it, surgery may be required.)

little extra effort, you can restore these muscles to the strength and elasticity needed to do the job.

What to Avoid

❏ Be wary of using a girdle. By binding and artificially supporting your abdomen, a girdle allows the muscles to become lazy and may further weaken them.

EXERCISE TECHNIQUES

(If you had a cesarean delivery, get your doctor's permission before starting abdominal exercises.)

If you exercised throughout your pregnancy, you have a head start on regaining your muscle tone. If not, it will take a little more time and work, but you *can* do it.

Leg Slides and Head Lifts can be done as soon as you like. Begin with Leg Slides, the easiest of the four, and gradually move on to the others in the order in which they appear here.

LEG SLIDES

Benefits: Tones abdominal muscles and leg muscles.

1. Lie flat on your back, with your knees bent.
2. Inhale and slide your left leg away from you until it is straight.
3. Exhale and slide your left leg back to a bent position.
4. Repeat with your right leg.
5. Do three to five repetitions with each leg several times a day.

Comments: Be sure to keep both your feet relaxed, not pointed or flexed, and keep them on the floor or bed—don't lift them.

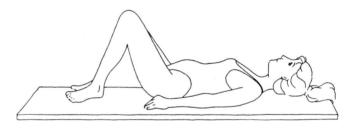

Leg Slides—Position 1

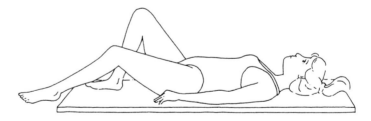

Leg Slides—Position 2

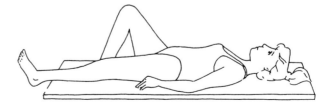

Leg Slides—Position 3

HEAD LIFTS

Benefits: Tones abdominal muscles and neck muscles.

1. Lie on your back with your knees bent.
2. Inhale and relax.
3. Exhale slowly while lifting your head off the floor or bed.
4. Inhale slowly and let your head back down.
5. Repeat five times.

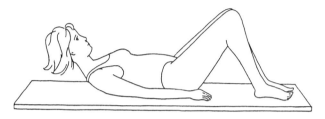

Head Lifts

Comments: Do the head lift slowly, without jerking. Concentrate on using your belly muscles to lift your head, and don't be alarmed if your abdomen begins to tremble. This is normal—it shows that your muscles are working hard. At first, lift your head only until the trembling starts, and then lower it again. As your muscles get stronger, try to keep your head raised for a slow count of three.

When your abdominal muscles no longer tremble with the Head Lift, you'll be ready for the next step:

SHOULDER LIFT

Benefits: Tones abdominal muscles and neck muscles.

1. Lie on your back with your knees bent.
2. Inhale and relax.
3. Exhale slowly while lifting your head and shoulders off the floor or bed.
4. Hold the position to a slow count of three.
5. Inhale slowly and let your head back down.

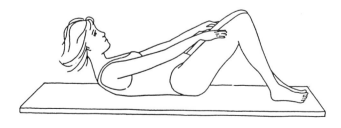

Shoulder Lifts

Comments: Lift your head and shoulders only to the point at which your muscles begin to tremble, or to a 45 degree angle, whichever comes first. Always exhale as you lift to help your muscles work more effectively.

This next exercise, the Abdominal Roll, should wait until you can do the Shoulder Lift easily and without trembling.

ABDOMINAL ROLL

Benefits: Tones abdominal muscles, and stimulates intestinal activity to relieve gas and constipation.

1. Stand with your feet about eighteen inches apart for support, and bend forward slightly from the waist. Brace your hands on your thighs.
2. Inhale.
3. Exhale as much air as possible, giving a grunt to get the last air out of your lungs.
4. Without inhaling again, pull your abdominal muscles in toward your spine as far as you can.
5. Inhale and relax your abdomen.
6. Exhale again, getting as much air out as possible.
7. Without inhaling, pull your abdominal muscles in and then push them back out so that they bulge in front. Try to do this three times without taking a breath.
8. Inhale and relax your muscles.
9. Take a few breaths and rest your lungs a bit.
10. Exhale all your air for the final step.
11. Without inhaling, pull your belly in as far as possible, and then pull the same muscles up toward your chest as far as possible, and follow by pushing them back out. (This should feel like you're rolling your belly in, up, and out. If you can't feel the muscles move upward, just imagine the movement as you try to do it. With practice it will happen.)

Comments: After you've mastered all the steps, you need do only the final one, repeating it three times each day. It may be hard to get the hang of the entire abdominal roll at first. Some women find that their muscles are so weak they can barely feel them pulling inward and they can't see this happen at all. The upward motion may be tricky at first, too. It seems that the only part no one has much trouble with is the outward motion. Unfortunately, all of us seem to be very good at bulging, but not so good at tightening.

(*See also* Abdominal Weakness, prenatal, page 8.)

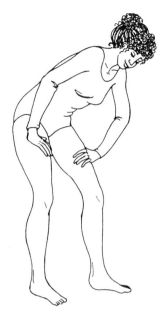
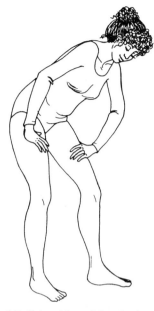

Abdominal Roll (pulling abdominal muscles in)   *Abdominal Roll (pushing abdominal muscles out)*

Baby Blues

"I can't explain how I feel to my husband. When the blues set in, I just hand him the baby and ask for his understanding. But it sure would feel great to have his arms around me."

About 50 to 80 percent of new moms experience "baby blues." It usually starts on the second or third day after the baby is born, and lasts no more than ten days. Symptoms include:

❏ Crying spells.   ❏ Decreased sex drive.
❏ Mood swings.   ❏ Worry about the baby.
❏ Anxiety.   ❏ Lack of confidence in
❏ Loneliness.   mothering ability.

PREVENTION

What to Do

❏ Begin during pregnancy to take steps to prevent baby blues by following the prevention and comfort measures described under "Mood Changes" on page 149 and by planning how you will arrange to follow through with the comfort measures listed on the next page after the baby is born.

Postpartum Depression: When It's More Than the Blues

Postpartum depression (PPD) is a "catch-all" term for a badly misunderstood syndrome. The experts disagree strongly about its definition, so I won't try to define it for you. But I *will* tell you how to recognize it and what to do about it.

Symptoms of PPD include:

- Inability to sleep, even when your baby is sleeping.
- Loss of appetite.
- Feelings of helplessness or loss of control.
- Over concern or no concern at all about your baby.
- Dislike or fear of touching your baby.
- Frightening thoughts about your baby.
- Little or no concern about your own appearance.
- Physical symptoms, such as difficulty breathing or palpitations.

If you have any of these symptoms, you should tell your husband, your birth attendant, and your childbirth educator how you feel. When caught early, PPD can be cured with medication and counseling. If the depression is severe or if depression is prolonged, temporary hospitalization may be necessary.

POSTPARTUM PSYCHOSIS

Postpartum psychosis is a rare condition that occurs in about 1 in every 1,000 new mothers. Psychosis means that the individual has lost touch with reality. This condition, which may or may not be preceded by depression, requires immediate psychiatric attention.

ABOUT YOUR BIRTH

You may feel disappointment or guilt if your birth didn't go as you'd hoped. If so, talk with your childbirth educator or with someone you love. And remember, giving birth is not a test; it's a labor of love. When it's over, what really counts is the love.

COMFORT

What to Do

- Get plenty of rest. Ask for help from family, neighbors, or friends, or hire a neighborhood teenager to watch your baby while you nap.
- Get some recreation every day. Plan outings with your baby, or ask someone to watch her while you go shopping, take a walk, attend an exercise class, or dine out with your husband.
- Eat well. Include plenty of whole grains, milk products, fresh fruits and vegetables, and protein-rich foods, such as fish, chicken, beef, cheese, and beans.
- Seek support. Tell your partner how you feel and ask for his help and support. Join a new mothers' group, or get to know other new moms at your church or workplace.
- Trust yourself. Remember, even without experience, most new parents do what's right for their baby.

What to Avoid

- Avoid over-analyzing your feelings. Baby blues are normal.
- Avoid trying to keep up the pace you did before the baby was born.

Give yourself some time to recuperate before resuming obligations to others.

❑ Avoid isolating yourself from family and friends. You need some private time, but you also need support and companionship.

A WORD TO THE NEW FATHER

If you're a new father whose wife has the baby blues, you're probably feeling confused about just what to do. It's hard for you to understand how a woman with a beautiful new baby in her arms could be so sad and weepy. You'll get a lot of advice about humoring her and letting her cry it out, but neither of these really helps. What your wife actually needs is lots of love and support and understanding—even if you don't *really* understand.

Baby blues often result in anxiety and loneliness, but they can also be caused by these same feelings. Most new moms feel unsure about their ability to take proper care of a newborn, and they're often quite sensitive to comments that they perceive as criticism of the way they're caring for the baby. The most important thing you can do for your wife is to let her know that you're there for her. Try to make sure she gets both the rest and recreation she needs, and, most important of all, show her that you care.

Oh! And don't be surprised if you get to feeling a little blue yourself. It happens to a lot of new dads. If it happens to you, follow the same advice for yourself that I've given to your wife.

Backache

Many of the causes of prenatal backaches disappear with the birth of the baby, but they may be replaced by new stresses on your body. For example, while you no longer have to carry all that extra weight everywhere you go, you still have a rapidly growing baby who needs to be carried everywhere *she* goes. Your back may also be feeling the results of all the work and strain of giving birth. If you had a long labor or a difficult delivery, your lower back may be tired and sore. Or you may have a lot of tension and discomfort in your upper back, neck, and shoulders from holding the pushing position for prolonged periods. Occasionally the baby's head is a little large for the mother's pelvis, or the child is born in a position that requires more space than the mother's birth canal allows. As a result, the mother's tailbone may end up bruised or cracked. This is an unusual problem and is more common in a *posterior presentation*, in which the back of the baby's head is against the mother's spine.

Some new mothers complain of pain after receiving spinal or epidural anesthesia. As with any injection, there may be some soreness after the effect of the anesthesia wears off, but it's unusual for the procedure to cause a persistent backache. If you're in pain and if you're sure that it's not just muscle soreness or a tired back, ask your doctor to check it for you.

PREVENTION

What to Do

❑ Protect your back while caring for your baby. She seems very small now and you may think that her weight isn't enough to matter, but she'll grow quickly and you should begin now to develop good habits that will let you care for her without straining your back. Here are several suggestions:

- While your baby is still too little to sit up, keep her crib mattress set at the highest level so that you don't have to reach down too far to work with her.
- When picking up your baby from a surface below the level of your waist, bend at your knees to reach for her. As you lift her to your level, use the strength of your legs to stand up.
- When bathing or diapering your baby, try to place her at a comfortable level that doesn't require you to lean over to reach her. If you don't have a changing table, use your kitchen or bathroom counter or your dining room table. Just place a pad or blanket on the surface, and be sure to keep one hand on the baby at all times so that she doesn't roll off.

❑ Use these abdominal strengthening exercises:

- Pelvic Tilt (page 10).
- Curl-Ups (page 12).
- Buttocks Curl (page 11).

What to Avoid

❑ Avoid exercises and movements that require you to arch your back, including double leg-lifts and full sit-ups.
❑ Avoid lifting heavy objects.

When It's More Than Just a Backache

If you have severe back pain or if you have pain in your tailbone that continues for more than three weeks after the birth, ask your birth attendant to check it for you. Your doctor may order an X-ray to see if your tailbone was cracked. This will give you a diagnosis, but unfortunately, there's not much you can do to speed the healing. In addition to the remedies above, the following suggestions can make you more comfortable while you're waiting:

What to Do

❑ When you have to sit, use a "do-nut," or rubber ring, to take some of the pressure off your tailbone. You can buy one at a drug store or medical supply house.

❑ Soak in warm water.

❑ Apply heat or ice to the painful area.

❑ Try the Kneeling Pelvic Tilt (page 19) and Knee-Chest (page 7) for temporary relief or pressure on your tailbone.

❑ Ask your doctor about pain medication.

What to Avoid

❑ Avoid lifting heavy objects.

❑ Avoid sitting for long periods.

❑ Avoid taking aspirin or ibuprofen during postpartum or while breastfeeding.

It can take several months for the discomfort to disappear, and some women are bothered by pain intermittently throughout their lives. If the bone was cracked or severely bruised, it may flare up with each pregnancy. There's also a chance of developing arthritis in this area.

❑ Avoid carrying your baby or anything else on your hip.

❑ Avoid prolonged sitting or standing.

COMFORT

What to Do

❑ Use Lower Back Massage (page 21). (This may help, even if the pain is due to a bruised or cracked tailbone. Notice that this pressure point is located at your waist level; *do not* apply pressure directly over the painful area.)

❑ Use Total Back Massage (page 23).

❑ Apply heat to relax and soothe tired, tense back muscles.

❑ Apply cold or heat to reduce the pain of a bruised or cracked tailbone.

❑ Rock in a rocking chair.

❑ Sleep with your knees bent or with your legs resting on a pillow.

What to Avoid

❑ See Prevention tips, "What to Avoid."

(*See also* Backache, prenatal, page 15.)

Breast Changes

During the past nine months your breasts underwent a number of changes as they prepared to nourish your baby. This process of change will continue after your baby is born. The normal process of producing milk, or *lactation,* began during pregnancy when your breasts started secreting colostrum. This clear, sticky liquid, with its natural antibodies, will provide the ideal nourishment for your baby for the first few days of life, until your milk comes in. This usually happens on the second, third, or fourth day. (The flow may be delayed if you were heavily medicated before or after the birth, if you had a cesarean delivery, or if you're sick.) Your milk will be a thin, pale white fluid and may have a slightly bluish tint. Despite its appearance, it's quite high in fats, proteins, and carbohydrates. In fact, it has just the right amount of everything your baby needs and wants.

When you produce milk, it's stored in the glands deep within your breasts. As your baby begins to suck, it signals certain tissues in your breasts to contract and to squeeze the milk toward your nipples and out into your baby's waiting mouth. Your breasts will feel warm and tingly as the milk comes in, or "lets down."

Engorged Breasts

When your milk first comes in, on the second, third, or fourth day after delivery, you may have more milk than your baby can drink. Your breasts may get so full that they become hot and swollen, or engorged.

COMFORT

What to Do

❑ Find your baby and start nursing. Her hunger is the best cure for your engorgement. If she won't nurse, it may be that your nipples are too swollen to fit in her mouth. You can help by using your own fingers to express the excess milk. Here's how:

- Place your thumb about one-and-a-half inches above your nipple and place your forefinger the same distance below it.
- Press in toward your chest and squeeze your thumb and finger together gently to express the milk out of the nipple. (Do not pull or squeeze your nipple.)
- Let the milk squirt right onto your baby's lips. After the first drop or two, she'll open her mouth. Just be careful to give her time to swallow. A few squirts may be all you need to bring your nipples down to a size your baby can manage.

❑ If you are *not* planning to breastfeed, apply an ice pack to reduce pain and swelling.

What to Avoid

❑ Avoid applying heat, which can make the swelling worse.

❑ If you do *not* plan to breastfeed, avoid expressing milk unless you absolutely must. Even then, let out only the few drops necessary to relieve the pressure. Each time your nipples are used to express milk by you or your baby, your body is stimulated to produce more milk. If you want to dry up your milk supply, this will only prolong your discomfort.

❑ Avoid narcotic pain relievers, which can cause a sleepy, unresponsive baby.

❑ Avoid aspirin or ibuprofen, both of which can cause bleeding. If you *must* take something, try an aspirin substitute.

Sore or Cracked Nipples

Although she seems tiny and weak, your newborn has powerful muscles in her mouth. For the first few weeks your nipples may feel sore, especially at the beginning of a feeding.

PREVENTION

What to Do

❑ When nursing, position your baby so that her entire body is facing you.

❏ When nursing, make sure your entire nipple and as much areola as possible is placed well back inside your baby's mouth and over the center of her tongue.

❏ If the baby is sucking incorrectly or nursing is painful, take her off the breast and start over. Check the suggestions for easier nursing on page 134. Doing it the right way is the best prevention for sore, cracked nipples.

What to Avoid

❏ Avoid breast pads with plastic-like coatings that do not allow moisture to evaporate.

❏ Avoid using soap, alcohol, or perfumed creams or lotions on your breasts.

❏ Avoid abruptly pulling your baby's mouth from your nipple. If she's nursing incorrectly, or if you need to stop the feeding, break the suction gently by slipping a finger inside your baby's mouth and pulling lightly on the inside of her cheek.

COMFORT

What to Do

❏ If you develop a cracked nipple, you may want to use a breast shield, but only as a temporary protection. It can reduce the amount of stimulation your nipples receive, which in turn can lower milk pro-duction.

❏ After each feeding, smooth a few drops of your own milk on your nipples to soothe them.

Clogged Duct

If your breasts are not emptied frequently and thoroughly, you may develop a clogged duct. This usually shows up as a small, sore, reddened lump. If it's not treated, it can become infected.

PREVENTION

What to Do

❏ Let your baby nurse twenty to thirty minutes every one-and-a-half to three hours.

❑ To be sure your breasts are emptied, either nurse the baby from only one breast at each feeding, or always start on the breast the baby nursed from last at the previous feeding. If you choose the second option, attach a safety pin to your bra strap to remind you which breast to start with at the next feeding.

❑ Change your baby's position occasionally so she can draw milk from all areas of your breast.

COMFORT

What to Do

❑ Nurse the baby longer and more often.

❑ Change your baby's position several times while nursing at the affected breast.

❑ After she finishes, hand-express any remaining milk.

❑ Until the duct clears, let your baby nurse first from this breast so that it will be more completely emptied.

Breast Infection

If your breast feels hot and tender and engorged, and if you have a headache or feel like you have the flu, you might have a breast infection, or *mastitis*. Report these symptoms to your birth attendant as soon as possible. She'll probably want you to take an antibiotic to clear up the infection.

PREVENTION

What to Do

❑ Follow the prevention and comfort measures listed for sore, cracked nipples and for clogged ducts.

COMFORT

What to Do

❑ Rest as much as possible.

❑ Keep allowing your baby to nurse from the infected breast.

Breastfeeding consultants usually encourage a mother to keep nursing from both breasts. They say not to worry about infecting your baby because she probably already has been exposed to the bacteria, and the antibiotic you're taking will be excreted in your milk.

❏ Apply moist heat to the affected area. (Some experts recommend an ice pack, so, if the heat doesn't seem to help, give it a try.)

❏ If you and your physician have decided to use an antibiotic to help clear up the infection, keep taking it according to directions until all the medicine is gone. Unless your doctor tells you otherwise, do not stop taking the medication until it's gone, even if the symptoms have disappeared.

Making Breastfeeding Easier for You and Your Baby

Breastfeeding is the method of choice for more than half of all new moms. Unfortunately, the most natural way to nourish your baby is not always the easiest to learn, and many mothers soon give up. Here are a few tips to make it easier:

❏ Nurse your baby as soon as possible after delivery. Early suckling helps stimulate your breasts to produce milk.

❏ Let your baby nurse twenty to thirty minutes every one-and-a-half to three hours. Offer both breasts at each feeding. (Experts used to recommend brief periods of nursing the first few days, but this may actually aggravate nipple problems and decrease your milk supply.)

❏ Nurse in a comfortable position, with your back, arms, and legs well supported. (A rocking chair is ideal, but if you don't have a chair that can support your arms comfortably while you hold your baby, try placing her in your lap, on top of several pillows.)

❏ Position your baby with her entire body facing you.

❏ Help your baby find your breast by stroking the cheek nearest you, or by using your nipple to tickle her lips. This will make her open her mouth. When she does, quickly place the nipple well back inside her mouth, while pulling her close to you.

❏ Be sure the nipple is centered over your baby's tongue, well back inside her mouth. She should be grasping most or all of the areola, the dark area surrounding your nipple.

❏ If the baby is sucking incorrectly or if nursing is painful, take her off the breast and start over. (Don't pull your nipple out of her mouth abruptly; break the suction first by slipping a finger inside her mouth and pulling gently on the inside of her cheek.)

Your milk supply will increase as your baby grows. It's the classic example of supply and demand. The following suggestions will help ensure a healthy supply and a satisfying experience for you and your baby:

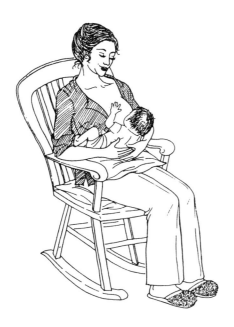

Breastfeeding While Sitting

❑ *Eat a well-balanced diet.* The average newborn requires about fifty calories daily for every pound of weight. This increases as she grows and becomes more active. If you're supplying all or part of her nutrition, you need to eat about 500 extra calories daily. To be sure they come from high quality foods, each day eat

four servings of milk products, four servings of fruits and vegetables, four servings of grains, and at least two or three servings of protein, such as fish, chicken, cheese, beans, or meat.

❑ *Drink at least eight glasses of liquids daily.* It takes liquid to make milk and, since everything for the milk has to come from you, you need to replenish your liquid supply daily. A good way to remember is to drink a glass of juice, water, or milk before or during each of the baby's feedings.

❑ *Get sufficient rest.* No matter how much milk you produce, it won't flow well if you're tired or tense. If necessary, put off other work in order to relax before you feed your baby. After all, nursing your child is extremely important work and the results can last a lifetime.

❑ *Be sure you and your baby are resting in a comfortable position.* If you're sitting up, your back and arms should be well supported. (A rocking chair is ideal.) If your arms or shoulders are tired, place several pillows in your lap and rest your baby on them. Just be sure she's high enough so that you don't have to lean over.

To nurse on your side, lie in bed with your baby resting on the mattress and facing you. (This is a good position if you've had a cesarean section.)

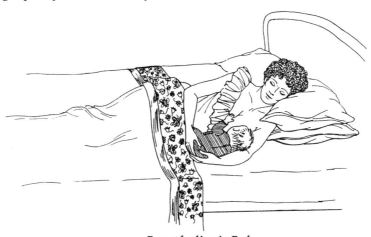

Breastfeeding in Bed

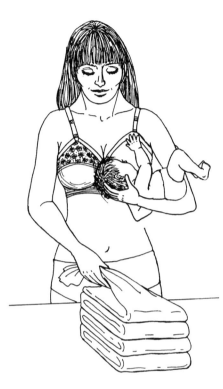

Breastfeeding With "Football Hold"

Another good position, called the "football hold," is a favorite with new fathers and it's ideal for the busy nursing mother. It's a great help if you're in the middle of something you can't stop and your baby is hungry. With one arm, hold your baby to your side so that your hand is under her head and your elbow is under her bottom. This leaves your other arm free to eat or answer the phone.

❑ *If your baby keeps nursing after most of your milk is gone, don't assume it means you don't have enough milk to satisfy her hunger.* When a bottlefeeding mother has problems feeding her baby, she wonders what's wrong with the baby. But when a breastfeeding mother has problems, she wonders what's wrong with her milk. Odds are, there's nothing wrong with your milk. Your baby is probably just satisfying her natural urge to suck. If you're comfortable with it, let her continue a while after each feeding. If you're not comfortable, or if your nipples are sore, consider using a pacifier to let her meet her sucking needs.

Breast Infection

See Breast Changes.

Constipation

You may have experienced frequent bouts with constipation while you were pregnant, and this problem may not disappear right away. There are two good reasons for being constipated right after the birth: you may have had diarrhea during early labor and you probably didn't eat during most of your labor. It makes sense that it may be several days before there's enough waste in your lower colon for a bowel movement. You may also be feeling the temporary after-effects of any pain medication or anesthesia you might have had during labor.

Another reason for constipation is that your rectum was under a great deal of pressure during the delivery, and the tissue around it may have become swollen. When these tissues return to normal, you will notice some relief. If you have hemorrhoids or perineal stitches, you may be afraid that it will hurt if you have a bowel movement. Unfortunately, your fear can aggravate the problem by giving any waste that is in your colon time to dry out. By the time you finally give in and go to the bathroom, the stool will be hard and will probably be about as uncomfortable to pass as you thought it would.

PREVENTION

What to Do

- ❏ See prevention measures listed under "Constipation" in the prenatal section of the Comfort Guide (page 36).
- ❏ Drink at least eight glasses of liquid daily.
- ❏ Eat whole grains and raw or lightly steamed fruits and vegetables.
- ❏ Exercise regularly. Walking, swimming, bicycling, and low impact exercises encourage your whole body, including your intestines, to work more efficiently.
- ❏ Use the Abdominal Roll (page 124), Pelvic Tilt (page 10), and Buttocks Curl (page 11) to help stimulate your intestines.
- ❏ Pay attention to your body's signals; if it says you need to go, then go.

What to Avoid

- ❏ Avoid putting off that first bowel movement. Use the relaxation techniques you learned in childbirth classes and don't worry about tearing your stitches—that would be awfully hard to do.

COMFORT

What to Do

- ❏ Follow the prevention measures listed above and in the prenatal section.
- ❏ Press your "Below Belly Button" to stimulate your intestines (see page 138).

What to Avoid

❑ Avoid medicated laxatives intended to stimulate your intestines. If you must take something, try one of the bulk laxative powders that you add to water.

MASSAGE TECHNIQUES

THE BELOW BELLY BUTTON

Benefit: Stimulates intestinal activity, and relieves gas and constipation. (Oriental philosophy credits this pressure point with improving energy and vitality and prolonging life.)

I like to think of this as a button I can push when I have a problem with constipation—sort of an extra "belly button." To find it:

1. Place your hand on your abdomen so that your thumb is at the lower edge of your umbilicus (belly button).
2. With your hand in this position, the pressure point is located in the midline of your body, just where your little finger is resting. Apply steady pressure here for a slow count of four.
3. Repeat this three times each morning and three times each evening.

(*See also* Hemorrhoids, prenatal, page 75; Hemorrhoids, postpartal, page 148; and Stitches, page 155.)

Depression

See Baby Blues.

Dizziness

After your baby is born, the nurse will caution you to ask for help the first time you get out of bed because you may feel dizzy when you stand up. Some women also have this problem when they sit up or when they rapidly change positions.

The lightheaded sensation is normal after the stress of childbirth and with all the sudden changes in your body. You abruptly lost a great deal of mass and weight from one area of your body, shifting your center of gravity. There are also changes in your bloodflow and in other fluids in your body. All these factors affect your balance.

PREVENTION

What to Do

❑ Move slowly and cautiously when rising from a lying or sitting position.

❑ Ask for help the first time or two you get up after giving birth.

❑ If you must be on your feet for more than a few minutes, keep moving. This keeps the blood pumping to your brain and reduces the chance of a dizzy spell.

What to Avoid

❑ Do not get out of bed by yourself if you have received a narcotic pain medication.

COMFORT

What to Do

❑ Lie down until the dizziness passes and then get up slowly.

❑ If lying down doesn't help, remain lying and elevate your legs on pillows to improve the bloodflow to your brain.

❑ If you're experiencing frequent dizziness, ask someone to stay in the room with you while you're holding your baby.

❑ Notify your doctor if you still have occasional dizzy spells after the first few days.

(*See also* Dizziness, prenatal, page 49; and Fainting, page 52.)

Fatigue

"No one ever told me how little sleep I'd get after the baby was born. Will my baby ever sleep all night through? Will I?"

What Happens When You Sleep

When you sleep, your mind and body go through cycles that last about forty-five minutes each. For a period you experience what is called REM, or rapid-eye-movement sleep, when you dream. Even a person who doesn't remember dreaming goes through several dream phases each night. This sleep phase helps restore energy and calm to your mind and emotions. The other cycle is one of deep sleep, during which your body is restored. If these cycles are interrupted, you won't get the same benefit you would receive from uninterrupted sleep, even if the total hours are equal. Each time you get up at night with the baby, you're breaking the natural sleep cycle and depriving yourself of the kind of rest you need.

KEEPING LIFE SIMPLE

After my first baby was born, I took a tour of my house and removed all the dust-collecting items that I could bear to put away for a while. An empty dresser or piano top is much easier to dust. By making the task easy I was able to do it more often, so I didn't feel depressed every time I passed a dirty piece of furniture. Besides, I found out that the dust and dirt would always wait for me, but my baby would keep on growing and changing. If I'd spent the extra time it takes to keep an immaculate house, I might have missed important and precious moments that I never could have retrieved.

When you were pregnant, you probably looked forward to the time when you'd lose all that weight, along with the backaches, swollen feet, and fatigue that went along with it. If so, you're probably disappointed to find that at least one of those problems—fatigue—is still a big problem. You put a lot of physical, emotional, and spiritual energy into helping your baby grow inside you and in bringing him out into the world. Even now your body is working hard to readjust to being "unpregnant." Along with these demands, you may be nursing a baby, which takes about 500 calories each day from your own nutritional reserves, along with a lot of emotional investment. Besides all this, you have to deal with your baby's unreliable schedule and his total dependence on you or some other adult for meeting his needs. Even if you catnap and accumulate a total of eight hours of sleep in a twenty-four-hour period, you're not getting the kind of rest you need to meet these new challenges.

PREVENTION & COMFORT

(Fatigue is a fact of life for every new mother, but the following measures can prevent excessive fatigue while making you feel more comfortable and energetic.)

What to Do

❑ Care for your own needs as well as you care for the needs of your baby. This means plenty of rest, nourishment, and stimulation. Here are a few tips:

- If possible, arrange for someone to help with chores, or consider serving sandwiches and convenience foods and letting other household chores slide for the next two weeks or so.

- Request that your friends and family not visit you for the first month. Invite only those with whom you feel comfortable without getting dressed up or making other special preparations.
- Devote part of at least one day a week to yourself. Leave the baby with someone for several hours and go shopping or take an exercise class or have your hair done. Do something that has nothing to do with babies or families. By being "selfish," there will be more of you to give to your family for the rest of the week.

❑ Exercise daily. I know you're tired and I know it's hard to believe that exercise will feel good, but it will! Moving your muscles stimulates your circulation, perks up your spirits, and is one of the best ways to counter fatigue. Put your baby in a stroller and take long, brisk walks. When he can hold his head up well, place him in a baby carrier and get going.

❑ Eat plenty of protein foods, such as meats, fish, eggs, cheese, and legumes, and continue taking an iron supplement. If you're nursing your baby, you'll need about 300-500 extra calories daily. If not, you still need extra protein and iron for a while to build up your nutritional reserves.

(*See also* Fatigue, prenatal, page 53; Mood Changes, page 83; Sexual Adjustments, page 151; and Weight, page 167.)

Fever

Fewer than 3 percent of all new mothers develop a postpartum infection, but it's important to report any symptoms to your birth attendant so he can decide if you need medical treatment.

PREVENTION

What to Do

❑ Drink plenty of fluids—at least eight glasses of water daily.
❑ See the Contents page of this book to locate ways of preventing illnesses that cause fever, such as breast and bladder infections.

Gas

WHAT ABOUT BREASTFEEDING?

If you're breastfeeding your baby, ask the pediatrician if it's alright to continue while you have fever. Your baby received many immunities from your colostrum, and if you're taking antibiotics, they'll be excreted in the milk and may prevent him from catching the infection, or may cure him if he already has it. Tell the doctor who is treating your fever that you're nursing, and tell the baby's doctor the type of infection you have and what medication you're taking.

COMFORT

What to Do

❑ Notify your birth attendant if you have a temperature above 100.4°F (38°C).
❑ Cool down fever by bathing in tepid water.
❑ Ask your partner to give you a rubdown with a mixture of one part alcohol to one part water. (Do not let your baby inhale this mixture.)
❑ If necessary, use an aspirin substitute to lower the fever. Follow package directions carefully, being sure not to take more than the recommended dosage.

What to Avoid

❑ *Do not take aspirin or ibuprofen* during the postpartum period. These medications can cause or increase bleeding.

(*See also* Breast Infection, page 133.)

Gas

Gas is sometimes a problem during postpartum, especially if you received a lot of pain medication or an epidural, spinal, or general anesthetic during labor. These drugs tend to temporarily paralyze or slow down your intestines, which can result in a build-up of gas.

PREVENTION

What to Avoid

❑ Avoid gas-producing foods, such as beans or strongly-flavored greens.
❑ Avoid constipation (see page 136).

COMFORT

What to Do

❑ Exercise regularly to stimulate your intestines. If you had a cesarean birth, or if your abdominal muscles feel especially weak, try Leg

Slides (page 122) and Head Lifts (page 123). Otherwise, use the Pelvic Tilt (page 10), Abdominal Roll (page 124), and Buttocks Curl (page 11).

❑ Use the "Below Belly Button" (page 138).

❑ Each morning, drink a glass of very warm water with the juice of half a lemon squeezed into it.

❑ Rock in a rocking chair for twenty or thirty minutes to help relieve gas pain.

What to Avoid

❑ Avoid prolonged use of commercial anti-gas preparations; they can cause constipation.

(*See also* Constipation, page 136.)

Grief

Pregnancy is supposed to have a happy ending. You may go through all sorts of changes and discomforts and pains in order to get through it but, when it's over, you're supposed to take home a beautiful, healthy baby. But it doesn't always happen this way. If you lost your baby to miscarriage, stillbirth, or neonatal death, you're probably going through one of the most difficult times in your life. I can't help you get rid of your grief in the confines of this book, but I *will* tell you how to start.

There are two things you need to know about grief:

1. *It's private.* You and your partner, and each friend or family member who is touched by your loss, will grieve in your own ways. You might need to express your grief through tears and you may feel an intense need to talk about it with someone who understands. But your partner might need to work out his grief differently. He may need to be alone, or he may feel he has to be calm and strong in order to help you through this. Try to give each other love and support, but also try to be patient and to respect one another's own way of handling your mutual loss.

2. *It's not predictable.* Many experts have outlined specific stages of grief. The problem is that no one grieves according to an outline. The best explanation of how grief progresses is given by Glen Davidson, author of "Understanding the Death of a Wished-for Child" (OGR Service Corp, 1979):

CHRONIC GRIEF

If your baby is alive, but not healthy, or if she has a birth defect, you're experiencing your own kind of grief. Many of the suggestions in this section will help you, but you'll find even more help from a local parents' support group. Your childbirth educator or birth attendant, or one of the nurses from the hospital where your baby was born, should be able to refer you to a local group of parents who have dealt or are dealing with a problem similar to yours. It may be difficult to go, at first, but you won't regret having done it.

Shock and numbness. At first nothing seems real. You don't believe that it really happened, and you don't want anyone to convince you it did.

Searching and yearning. This is when you feel the loss most deeply. You may have an intense need to know what happened to cause you to lose your baby. You may spend a lot of time thinking and talking and dreaming about your baby. You may feel angry, or guilty, or restless, or just confused.

Disorientation. You may feel depressed, but may try to make others think that you're okay. Or you may feel disorganized or weak and listless and you may not feel like doing anything at all.

Reorganization. It can take many months to reach this stage when you feel a sense of freedom and renewed energy. You make decisions more easily and carry on your daily tasks much as you did before you were pregnant. You still remember your baby, and you still wish she was alive and well and in your arms, but you look forward to the future and to other happy times that lie ahead.

You won't go through these stages at a set pace, and you won't necessarily go through them one at a time. Your feelings may change from day to day or even from minute to minute, and you may go back and forth between stages until you reach "Reorganization." Even then, you'll probably feel a sudden sadness or wistfulness at certain anniversary dates, such as the date you first learned you were pregnant or the date your baby was born.

SPIRITUAL STRENGTH

Many couples whom I've counseled have sought and found comfort and peace in their personal faith. For them, and perhaps for you, spiritual guidance can be one of the most important sources of help. I've also gained a great deal of peace from an anonymous verse on a plaque that hung in my office for many years:

"Sometimes the Lord calms the storm; sometimes He lets the storm rage, and calms His child."

COMFORT

(The following suggestions apply to both you and your partner.)

What to Do

☐ Talk with your spouse. Give each other plenty of love and support.

☐ Find someone, other than your spouse, to whom you can talk without fear of judgment—someone who will listen but will not offer advice that may not be right for you.

☐ Let yourselves cry for a while, but let yourselves hope, too.

☐ Take care of yourselves physically. Get plenty of rest and good nutrition and try to get some exercise or recreation several times a week.

☐ Insulate yourselves with the love of a few close friends or relatives until you feel stronger.

❑ Be patient with yourself and your spouse. Don't try to resume all your usual work and activities before you're ready. Some work can be therapeutic, but too much will block out those important, but painful, thoughts that must be dealt with for a while.

❑ Find out exactly what caused your baby's death and whether there's any way to prevent its repetition.

❑ Do what *you* want to about funeral or memorial service arrangements. Don't let the hospital or your family pressure you into anything with which you don't feel comfortable.

❑ Give your baby a name. This will give her a more definite and permanent place in your family and its history. And don't be afraid to use her name when talking about her.

❑ When help is offered, take it. Give friends specific suggestions for ways they can help; for example, ask someone to drop off your laundry or pick up your groceries or bring a casserole. Or maybe you just want someone who will listen.

❑ Talk to your birth attendant and childbirth educator about a local support group for grieving parents. And talk with your minister, priest, or rabbi. Your loss is physical and emotional, but it's also deeply spiritual.

What to Avoid

❑ Avoid trying to hold everything inside.

❑ Avoid worrying about protecting others' feelings; focus on your own and on your partner's for now.

❑ Avoid throwing yourself into your work or a project to keep from thinking about your baby.

❑ Avoid conceiving another child right away. Give yourself time to mourn and say goodbye to this baby.

Hair Changes

As your hormones return to a nonpregnant level, your hair will resume its natural state, as well. This means that the hairs you didn't lose during pregnancy will begin falling out. This may begin a few weeks after the birth and continue for several weeks. The amount and duration of hair loss varies among women, but most will replace the lost hairs within a few months. Meanwhile, a professional hairdresser can help you find an attractive way to arrange your hair.

PREVENTION

What to Do

- ❑ Continue following the suggestions for prenatal hair care on page 64.
- ❑ Continue taking prenatal vitamins for the next few months.

What to Avoid

- ❑ Avoid overworking or overheating your hair.

(*See also* Hair, prenatal, page 64.)

Headaches

Many women find that they have fewer headaches after the baby is born; others say that's when the headaches begin. The most common cause of postpartal headaches is probably a combination of tension and fatigue. You'll find remedies for postpartum fatigue on page 139 and for mood changes on page 149.

"Spinal Headaches"

Perhaps the most severe form of postpartal headache is the "spinal headache." This is more common after a spinal anesthesia, such as a saddle block, but it can also happen after an epidural. It's caused when some of the fluid in the spinal canal leaks out through the hole left by the needle. Women usually use words like "severe," "blinding," and "stabbing" to describe the pain of this headache. It may also be accompanied by stiffness in the neck, which may be due to the tension caused by continuous pain. The headache will probably persist until the spinal fluid has replaced itself. The time varies, but by the end of the second week most women report no more pain.

For most women, it takes strong drugs to relieve this pain. Your doctor may offer to prescribe a narcotic or a sedative, or a combination. But these can make you sleepy and can slow down your recovery, and, if you're breastfeeding, they will reach your baby. That's why it's always best to try natural remedies first. The most helpful ones will be the pressure and cold techniques described for prenatal migraine headache (page 65). Notify your doctor if you have a headache or neck stiffness accompanied by fever.

The first days and weeks of motherhood usually are thought of as being full of joy and fulfillment. A persistent headache can wear you down and make you doubt the whole idea of the beauty of being a mother. Keep in mind that this will pass. Meanwhile, apply your own knowledge and abilities to make yourself as comfortable as possible.

PREVENTION

What to Do

❑ Take time to take care of yourself. Your body and mind are parts of the same whole; when one is fatigued the other is, too. Emotional exhaustion leads to physical exhaustion, along with symptoms like headaches. Now, when you're so busy adjusting to a new life and a new lifestyle, is the time to be kind to yourself. Exercise or take a walk several times a day, rest when you can, and be patient with yourself. Soon things will return to a more normal state.

What to Avoid

❑ Avoid trying to keep up an image of the super-mother/super-wife. There's no such person.
❑ Avoid the triggers listed on page 66 if you are prone to migraines.

COMFORT

What to Do

❑ Use any or all of the following:

- Temple Massage (page 69).
- Upper Neck Massage (page 69).
- Shoulder Massage (page 22).
- Facial Massage (page 70).
- Soothing Touch Massage (page 69).

❑ Use Sequential Relaxation (page 72).
❑ Use the Relaxation Countdown (page 73).
❑ Apply a cold compress to the painful area. (If the headache is not a migraine, you may use either a hot or cold compress.)
❑ Drink a soothing cup of herbal tea.
❑ Have a glass of milk with cookies or crackers. (The tryptophan in the

milk, combined with the carbohydrates in the cookies or crackers, produces a relaxing, soothing effect.)

What to Avoid

❏ *Do not take aspirin or ibuprofen* during postpartum. If you need pain medication, try an aspirin substitute.
❏ Avoid applying heat to your head if you have a migraine headache.

(*See also* Headaches, prenatal, page 65; Fatigue, postpartal, page 139; and Mood Changes, postpartal, page 149.)

Hemorrhoids

Whether or not you noticed any hemorrhoids during pregnancy, you may have some now. As you strained and pushed to deliver your baby, the pressure may have caused internal hemorrhoids to protrude from your rectum. These varicose veins, or piles, will look like a pink cauliflower bud sitting on the edge of your rectum. Hemorrhoids can itch and hurt, and they may also bleed.

Be sure to notify your birth attendant if the hemorrhoids bleed. They'll probably decrease in size after a while, and may even seem to disappear completely, but once you've developed hemorrhoids, you're likely to have recurrences in other pregnancies and later in life. If hemorrhoids become a chronic and bothersome problem, your doctor may refer you to a surgeon for their removal.

PREVENTION

What to Do

❏ Drink eight glasses of fluid daily.
❏ Include at least two servings each of whole grains and raw fruits or vegetables in your daily diet.
❏ Exercise regularly.
❏ If you did not develop hemorrhoids during pregnancy and if none were discovered during or after the birth, you probably won't develop them any time soon. But, since they are a common problem, it's wise to make the prevention tips listed in the prenatal section a lifetime habit.

COMFORT

What to Do

- ❑ Use the Kegel exercise (page 28).
- ❑ Soak in a tub of very warm water.
- ❑ When trying to have a bowel movement, place your feet on a small stool or box to provide better leverage and prevent excess straining.
- ❑ For painful external hemorrhoids, elevate your hips using the Knee-Chest position or by lying on your back and placing one or two pillows under your hips. While in this position, apply cotton balls soaked in cold witch hazel to your rectum.
- ❑ Consult your birth attendant or family physician for medical advice regarding external or bleeding hemorrhoids.

(*See also* Constipation, prenatal, page 36; Constipation, postpartal, page 136; Hemorrhoids, prenatal, page 75; and Varicose Veins, page 112.)

Mastitis

See Breast Changes.

Mood Changes

Remember those mood swings you had when you were pregnant? Well, in case you haven't already figured it out, they're not over yet. Lots of new moms experience mood swings. Although they can make it more difficult to enjoy getting to know your baby, they're a natural response to the fatigue you're probably feeling, as well as all the physical and emotional changes you've gone through in the past few months. Hormones play a major role in how you feel and in how you react to different situations. After your baby was born and the placenta detached from the uterine wall, your body began undergoing dramatic shifts in hormonal levels, and it may take a few weeks to adjust to these changes.

Besides physical changes, having a baby can make a big difference in your life and in your relationship with your husband and, in many

Bonding: It's Not Another Name for Glue

Many women expect to feel an overwhelming sense of love for their baby the minute he's born, and some of them do. But for others it takes a little longer for this love to develop. Called "bonding," the process of falling in love with your baby, and his falling in love with you, depends on a number of factors. The most important one is that you and your baby need to be together, seeing and feeling and smelling one another. But if you had a cesarean birth, you may have felt groggy the first day or two, making it difficult to begin relating to your child. And, if your baby was premature or needed intensive care, you probably weren't able to spend as much time as you'd hoped holding and nursing him.

Even if everything went great, there are a number of reasons that bonding may be delayed. For example, just as adults can be outgoing or shy, babies can be, too. If your baby isn't the outgoing type, he may not respond as readily at first to your attempts to communicate as another baby might.

Another reason for delayed bonding is something called a "fantasy baby." During pregnancy you probably imagined what your baby would look like, and, as happens with most expectant mothers, you may have fallen in love with this fantasy baby. Now that he's actually here, he's probably quite different from your fantasy, and you may feel disappointed or surprised by this unexpected result. You may also feel a bit guilty for reacting this way. But, no matter what the reason for the delay, you and your baby will eventually fall in love with another. It may happen all at once, with your baby's first smile or his first real tears. Or it may happen gradually, as your baby's personality emerges and you and he discover what makes each other special. And, when it does happen, you'll know it was worth the wait.

cases, with your own parents. Most people find themselves feeling a bit confused and ambivalent about it all. These feelings usually fade as you adjust gradually to your new role as a mother and your body adjusts to its nonpregnant state.

PREVENTION

What to Do

❏ Take care of yourself. A well-balanced diet, exercise, and rest are important in preventing and relieving moodiness. Your brain is controlled by a number of chemical and hormonal substances, whose production depends on a good supply of blood and oxygen and nutrients. The most effective way to provide these is through exercise, which stimulates your circulation; rest, which lets your body repair itself and recover its energies; and good nutrition, which supplies your central nervous system with what it needs to maintain a healthy emotional balance. (Continue your prenatal vitamins for the next few months to ensure that you're getting all the nutrients needed.)

❑ See prevention tips for prenatal mood changes on page 149.

COMFORT

What to Do

❑ Use the following to help restore calm and a sense of emotional balance and control:

- Temple Massage (page 69).
- Upper Neck Massage (page 69).

❑ Use the following when you want to gain control of your emotions quickly:

- Soothing Touch (page 69).
- Sequential Relaxation (page 72).
- Relaxation Countdown (page 73).

❑ Seek support. Talk with your husband, your mom, your friends, or other new mothers. Call your childbirth educator and ask for the number of a local mothers' support group.

❑ Seek solace. Spend some quiet time with yourself. Ask someone to watch your baby while you take a walk or go to the library. When your baby is sleeping, take a few minutes to meditate or pray or read the Bible or another book that has helped you before.

Sexual Adjustments

One of the most frequently asked questions in the last childbirth class of the series is, "How soon after birth can we resume our normal sex life?"

It's usually safe to have intercourse after the postpartum vaginal discharge (lochia) stops. This usually happens about three weeks after the baby is born. Of course, if you had a difficult pregnancy or a complicated birth or postpartum, you should rely on your own birth attendant's advice regarding sexual activity.

For many couples the changes of pregnancy have upset the balance in their relationship, and they're counting on things returning to normal soon after the baby is born. While your love life might return to normal right away, many couples find their sexual desires temporarily altered after the birth. You or your husband may also find yourself so involved in your new role as parent that you temporarily forget your role as spouse and lover. Suddenly it seems that your whole world is made up of diapers and bottles and crib sheets. If this describes your life right now, you're probably wondering if you'll ever again be interested in sex and, if so, will you ever find time for it? The answer is most likely a resounding "Yes." Right now you're working very hard to adapt to a new role. If this is your first baby, you may be confounded by all the new demands on you. If this is not your first, you may be confused about just how you're going to organize yourself to meet the needs of your family. What's happening to you is the same thing that often happens when someone takes on a new and demanding position. When someone receives a promotion that brings with it a tremendous amount of responsibility, she may throw herself into the work so completely that she forgets everything else for a while. But, once that individual feels confident in the new role, she finds the time to stop and look around and realize that she's missing other important aspects of life. Given time, you'll learn how to cope with your new role, and within weeks, you probably will be devoting as much of yourself to your other roles, such as wife, daughter, and person, as you are giving now to your role as mother.

Several other problems that might interfere with your relationship are fatigue, fear of pain, concern over how the baby may have changed

Don't Forget the Birth Control

Decide together what you're going to do about birth control, and then do it. This will get rid of any fears you have of becoming pregnant again. Even if you had a perfect pregnancy and a great birth, and even if your baby is terrific, you're not emotionally or physically ready to do it again right now. You should wait at least a year after the birth before conceiving again, so that your body can build its nutritional reserves back to a level that will support a healthy pregnancy. If you're nursing your baby, begin counting this year from the time you wean him.

The lochia, or vaginal discharge, will last about three weeks. When this stops, your system will go back to its normal cycle of preparing each month for pregnancy. This means you can ovulate within two weeks after the lochia stops. Your first period will follow in another two weeks or so. In other words, do not wait for a period before you begin to practice birth control. Ovulation precedes menstruation. If you nurse your baby, your ovulation may be delayed, but this is not a reliable method of birth control.

Ask your doctor or childbirth educator about various methods of contraception. Be sure to look into the natural methods, such as rhythm and Billings ovulation method. When combined, these two natural methods can be extremely reliable.

your feelings for one another, and fear of conceiving again before you're ready. These are common concerns for new parents, and there are a variety of ways to deal with them.

PREVENTION & COMFORT

What to Do

❏ Reduce the possibility that intercourse may be uncomfortable by using these remedies:

- Find a position that avoids placing too much pressure on the woman's perineum. Lie side by side, facing one another, or let the man lie on his back with the woman on top of him. (This last position lets her control both the direction and the amount of pressure and may give her more confidence so she can relax and enjoy the experience.)

- Use a lubricant to make intercourse more comfortable. You'll have less vaginal lubrication in the weeks after the birth and while you're nursing. You or your husband can apply a water-soluble lubricant to the perineum, massaging it in to gently relax and stretch the area. You'll also want extra lubrication either inside the vagina or on the penis.

- Take a nice, long soak in warm water before having intercourse. This will relax you and will soothe and soften your perineal area.

❏ Practice the Kegel (page 28) frequently throughout the day to help your perineal tissues regain their elasticity.

❏ Before you begin, take turns giving one another a Total Back Massage (page 23) to help you both relax. Or use any of the relaxation techniques described in this book. (Remember what you learned in childbirth classes—tension increases pain.)

❏ Be patient with one another. Take it slowly and easily, letting your partner know what feels good and what does not.

❏ If you're breastfeeding, your nipples may leak, or even squirt, milk when you're aroused. Before having intercourse, nurse your baby or express your milk into a bottle for later nursing. If leaking still occurs, and if it bothers you or your husband, you may want to wear a bra with nursing pads or cover yourself with a towel.

(*See also* Baby Blues, page 125; Fatigue, page 139; Mood Changes, postpartal, page 149; Sexual Adjustments, prenatal, page 98; and Stitches, page 155.)

Shakes

Many new mothers begin to shiver right after the baby is born. Your entire body may quiver uncontrollably. This can be scary, but it is a normal reaction to the tremendous amount of effort and energy you exerted in giving birth. Remember, too, that you've just lost a great deal of body heat: your baby, placenta, and amniotic fluid made up about twelve pounds of tissue that held a constant temperature of 98.6°F. And, to make matters worse, hospital delivery rooms are famous for their cold temperatures. Within an hour the problem will probably be gone, but you may experience intermittent episodes of shakes for several days after the birth.

COMFORT

What to Do

❏ Ask for a warm blanket. Many hospitals keep a stack of blankets in a warmer. The nurse will probably cover you with one of these, but if she forgets, don't hesitate to ask for one.

❏ Rest and keep warm and it will pass.

❏ Remind yourself that this is normal and temporary.

❏ Ask your partner to apply the Soothing Touch (page 69) to help you remain calm and relaxed.

❏ Do your favorite slow-breathing relaxation technique, using your baby's eyes for a focal point.

Shoulder Pain

Shoulder pain may occur after a cesarean or vaginal delivery, but for different reasons. If you had a cesarean birth, you may feel pain in one shoulder. This is caused by air that entered your abdominal cavity during surgery. The air places pressure on your diaphragm, just under your lungs, but due to the structure of the nerves, the pain is often referred to the shoulder. It will take several days for the air to be absorbed and removed by your body's own processes.

After a vaginal delivery, your shoulders may ache because of the tension and effort of labor and delivery. This is especially true if you had to push for a long time, or if you're one of many women who respond to each contraction by tensing their shoulders or sitting up a bit in the bed. It will take several days for your strained shoulder muscles to recover from this experience.

COMFORT

What to Do

❑ Use the Forward Bend (page 20) and Shoulder Circles (page 20) to reduce shoulder pain caused by muscle soreness.

❑ Use Shoulder Massage (page 22) or Total Back Massage (page 23) to relieve shoulder pain of either kind. If you have no one to help you, use your own fingers or a blunt object to apply pressure on the first shoulder point (page 22). At this highest point on your shoulder, you'll probably feel a knot or fibrous area. This is where you should use your finger or thumb to apply pressure. You'll know you have the right spot if, when you apply pressure, it feels tender.

❑ Apply heat or cold to the highest point on your shoulder (see Shoulder Massage, above and on page 21.)

❑ Sit in a rocking chair and rock gently to help relieve shoulder pain due to air or muscle soreness.

(*See also* Backache, prenatal, page 15; and Backache, postpartal, page 127.)

Stitches, Perineal and Abdominal

Perineal Stitches

One of the most common postpartum complaints is pain in the area of the episiotomy. This surgical procedure is often done to allow more room for the baby's head during birth. There's a great deal of controversy over the necessity of routinely cutting the perineum, or the area between the vagina and the rectal opening, in order to enlarge the birth canal. Many women would not need one if they were able to give birth at their own pace and in a sitting or squatting position and if perineal massage were done. The purpose of this section, however, is not to discuss the pros and cons of routine episiotomy, but to help you deal with any discomfort that may arise if you had one or if you had a vag-inal or perineal laceration or tear.

Although the incision or tear is usually small, it occasionally involves deeper tissue and, rarely, may affect the rectal muscles or, in the case of a bad tear, the cervix. But, big or small, the cut almost always causes some discomfort as it heals. Some new mothers complain that their stitches are far more uncomfortable than the labor and delivery; others say they feel little or no pain from the stitches. Most fall somewhere in between these two extremes.

The suture used in repairing the perineum is usually the absorbable type, so it won't need to be removed later. As the stitches heal and absorb, you may find a piece of suture on your sanitary pad. This doesn't mean that the stitches are broken; it means they're healing.

COMFORT

What to Do

- ❏ Use the Kegel exercise (page 28). It will speed your healing by increasing the blood flow to the area and restoring the elasticity of the perineal muscles. Do this simple tightening and releasing exercise as often as you think of it. Contract the muscles of your perineum as though you are trying to hold back urine or gas. Hold for about five seconds and then release. Try to begin this exercise while the area is still numb from the anesthesia that was used for the suturing. This will make it easier to do later.
- ❏ Soak in very warm water.
- ❏ Use a moistened towelette to clean yourself after going to the bathroom. These are designed for hemorrhoid patients or new mothers to use instead of toilet paper, and are available at drug and grocery stores.
- ❏ Use a squeeze bottle to spray warm water on your perineum after going to the bathroom.
- ❏ If your birth attendant prescribed an anesthetic spray, use it.
- ❏ If you had a very large episiotomy or a severe tear, or if your stitches are very uncomfortable for some other reason, your doctor may prescribe a stronger pain reliever. If you're breastfeeding, keep in mind that most drugs are excreted in the milk.
- ❏ If you have a great deal of discomfort after leaving the hospital,

may want to rent or purchase an inflatable rubber ring, or do-nut, from a pharmacy or medical supply house. This allows you to sit down without putting pressure on the stitches.

What to Avoid

❏ Avoid taking aspirin or ibuprofen during postpartum or while nursing. If you need something, try an aspirin substitute.

❏ Avoid applying heat to perineum if area is swollen. Consult your birth attendant.

(*See also* Constipation, postpartal, page 136.)

Abdominal Stitches

Most cesarean births are done through a *transverse*, or horizontal, incision just at or above the pubic hairline. But, if yours was an emergency cesarean, or your baby was in a breech position, you might have a *classic*, or vertical, incision running from just below the umbilicus down to the pubic area. (The incision made in your uterus is almost always low and transverse, even if the skin incision is not.) The stitches used to repair your uterus, as well as the tissue layers beneath your skin, are absorbable. As these areas heal, the stitches will dissolve and be absorbed by your body. The skin incision is usually repaired with clips, or staples, or with a non-absorbable threadlike material. Your doctor may remove these before you leave the hospital, or later in her office. Afterward, she may apply thin strips of tape to the incision for added protection. If you haven't been able to bathe or shower yet, you'll probably be allowed to do so after the stitches are removed. Until then, you may have to rely on sponge baths.

Your doctor will order a potent pain medication, which will probably be available by injection every four hours or so during the first twenty-four or forty-eight hours. Later, as the pain lessens, you'll receive pain medication in a pill or capsule. Although the medication will make you more comfortable, it may also make you drowsy or dizzy, so again, be sure to ask for help before getting out of bed.

By the end of the first week, your pain should be greatly diminished and you probably won't require prescription medication for it. The skin that immediately surrounds the scar will feel numb, but you may continue to experience occasional soreness or burning in the incision itself for about six to eight weeks.

COMFORT

What to Do

❏ Help your abdominal muscles regain elasticity by letting them gently stretch several times a day. To do this, lie flat in bed for ten or fifteen minutes using relaxation breathing to relax your abdomen and ease the discomfort.

❏ Stand as straight as possible when you walk to reduce the length of time your muscles are sore.

❏ Move slowly for the first few days to reduce pain associated with activity.

❏ Cross one or both arms over your lower abdomen to help brace the incision when you walk, turn over, or cough.

❏ In the hospital, keep the bedrails up and use them for support when you turn over.

❏ Ask that a trapeze be placed over your bed. This metal triangle hangs from a bar over the bed and allows you to hold on to it as you move.

❏ Use relaxation to lessen the pain of moving. You'll probably feel a sharp pain around the incision as you begin to move. The injured muscles and nerves are extra sensitive right now, and they tend to create painful spasms whenever stimulated. If you respond by tensing up, it will only make matters worse.

To stop the spasms, try these:

• As soon as you feel the spasm start, take a deep sigh, releasing your abdominal muscles as you let it out. If you're sitting or standing when a spasm occurs, lean forward at the waist and let your muscles go limp. Then, close your eyes, take a sigh, and start breathing slowly and rhythmically, consciously releasing your abdominal muscles with each exhalation.

• If you feel a spasm begin when you're trying to turn over, let yourself go completely limp. Close your eyes gently and breathe slowly and deliberately. With each exhalation feel the abdominal muscles let go and loosen and relax. (The Balloon relaxation technique on page 163 is excellent here.)

• If a nurse is helping you to turn or get up, explain first that you will be using relaxation to ease any pain. If you are trying to sit up or get out of bed, let the nurse know that if you feel a muscle spasm start you will lean against her for support. If the nurse is not with you, and you have permission to get up alone, always keep your over-the-bed tray in a locked position and place a pillow on it. You can use this for support.

❑ Ask your doctor when you may get the stitches wet. When he says it's okay, soak in warm water for comfort.

❑ If you take a prescription pain reliever, ask for help before getting out of bed. If it's a strong medication or one that makes you sleepy, ask someone to stay with you while the baby is in the room.

What to Avoid

❑ Avoid favoring the stitches more than is necessary. At first, any activity tends to increase the pain, and you may be tempted to move as little as possible. But it's important to remember that moving about and walking help to speed your recovery and prevent complications. You may be tempted to bend forward whenever you're standing or walking, and to rest in a semi-sitting position with your knees bent when you're in bed. These postures are more comfortable because they ease the pull on your stitches. But they can slow down your progress by over-pampering the injured muscles.

❑ Avoid wearing pants or skirts with a front zipper or any other clothing that places uncomfortable pressure on the scar.

❑ Avoid taking aspirin or ibuprofen during postpartum or while breastfeeding.

(*See also* Abdominal Weakness, page 120; and Fatigue, postpartal, page 139.)

Sweating

Remember all that fluid retention you had when you were pregnant? Now that the pregnancy is over, you no longer need this added fluid, so your body will begin immediately to release it in the form of urine and perspiration. During the first week or so after giving birth, you may be surprised at the amount of sweat your body produces as it seeks to rid itself of this fluid. Within a few days your face will lose much of its puffiness, as will your legs, feet, and hands. You may even wake up at night to find your bed sheets soaked with sweat. This heavy sweating, called *diaphoresis,* is normal during this early postpartum time. You can't prevent it, nor would you want to. It's essential that your body be allowed to take care of its needs in this way.

COMFORT

What to Do

- ❑ Shower daily with a mild deodorant soap. (If you're nursing your baby, do not wash your breasts with soap—it will dry your nipples and make them more vulnerable to cracking.)
- ❑ If excess sweating leaves your hair extra oily, shampoo each day, applying shampoo only once. Be sure to rinse well, and if you use heat instruments to dry or set your hair, use a conditioner.
- ❑ After bathing or showering, apply corn starch or baby powder to help keep you comfortable and fresh.

What to Avoid

- ❑ Avoid using a feminine hygiene spray. These products, meant to prevent vaginal odor, can irritate the delicate tissues and are totally unnecessary if you follow good hygiene practices.

(*See also* Hair Changes, prenatal, page 64; Hair Changes, postpartal, page 145; and Vaginal Discharge, page 165.)

Urinary Difficulty

Some women find it difficult to urinate on the first day or two after giving birth. You're more likely to have this problem if a spinal or epidural anesthesia was used, or if a large baby or a difficult delivery caused swelling and bruising of the tissue around your bladder and urethra. This problem is almost always temporary. As soon as the anesthesia has fully worn off, or when the swelling subsides, your system should be back to normal. If you're still unable to urinate eight to twelve hours after the birth, a nurse will probably empty your bladder for you by inserting a narrow, flexible tube, called a catheter, through the urethra (the urinary opening) and into your bladder. Urine will pass quickly through the tube into a container, and then the tube will be removed. After that, you'll probably be able to urinate on your own.

If yours was a cesarean delivery, you probably had a Foley, or indwelling, catheter placed in your bladder before the surgery. It may remain in place for about twenty-four hours. This helps prevent bladder damage during the surgery, and keeps you from having to get up often after the operation. While the Foley is in place, you may be disturbed by an urge to urinate. This urgency is due to the pressure of the catheter on the nerves of your bladder. Don't worry—you won't have an accident; your bladder is being emptied by the tube and you only need to relax and let it happen. When the indwelling catheter is removed, the nurse will use a syringe to deflate the small, water-filled balloon that held the catheter inside your bladder, preventing it from slipping out. After this is done, the tube slips out easily. This procedure should not be uncomfortable and takes only a few minutes. It's fairly common to have some difficulty urinating at first after the Foley catheter is removed.

Whether or not you had a catheter inserted, the following remedies will help you urinate more easily.

COMFORT

What to Do

❑ Help your muscles relax by practicing your favorite slow-breathing relaxation technique while on the toilet. The Balloon (page 163) is a good one for this purpose.

❑ Sit in a tub of warm water and try to urinate into the water.

❑ Use a squeeze bottle to spray warm water over your urethra while you're on the toilet.

❑ Dangle your fingers in a glass of water while on the toilet. It may help if you pour warm water over your urethral opening as you sit on the toilet.

❑ Drink plenty of liquids, especially if you had a catheter. This will help prevent a bladder infection, which is more common among women who have been catheterized.

Uterine Involution

Immediately after your baby was born the top of your uterus, the *fundus,* was about at the level of your umbilicus. On the first day, if you press deeply into your abdomen near your belly button, you can feel the fundus. It should be about the size and firmness of a grapefruit. It feels hard because it's contracting in order to slow down the bleeding and help your uterus return to its normal size. This process, called *involution,* takes several weeks. Although your uterus will never be as

Fundal Massage

The involution process is generally spontaneous, but if you had a medicated birth or if you're not breastfeeding, your uterus may need a little help. But, even if you had a natural childbirth and are breastfeeding, your uterus will relax a little, at first. That's why, on the day after your baby's birth, you may not feel the fundus where it was the day before, at the level of your umbilicus. If so, move your hand up a bit and press deeply. If you still don't feel the hard, round top of your uterus, massage in a circular motion about two inches above your navel (see figure below). This should stimulate your uterus to contract and you'll feel the fundus hardening under your fingers.

To encourage involution and prevent excess bleeding, the postpartum nurse will massage your fundus several times a day. You can help speed your recovery by doing this yourself about every four hours during the day. If it's uncomfortable, try the relaxation techniques described in this section.

At first, you may notice an increase in vaginal bleeding during or right after massage. This is because the contractions brought on by the massage force out a gush of lochia, the normal postpartum vaginal discharge. This is a good sign that your massage is effective.

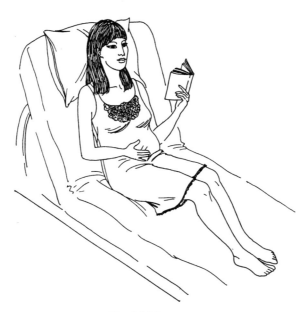

Fundal Massage

small as it was before it carried a baby, it will shrink considerably. By the time you go for your six weeks exam, it will have shrunk small enough to be hidden by your pubic bone.

You may notice mild contractions as the *involution* process occurs. They usually occur sporadically and are noticeable for only the first few days after the birth. These contractions are often referred to as after-pains, although most women don't find them painful. I have met some new moms however, who had considerable discomfort. Most of these women were nursing mothers or had already had a previous birth. If you're nursing, you'll have more and stronger afterpains because your infant's suckling stimulates the release of the hormone *oxytocin*, which, in turn, stimulates your uterus to contract. (This is only one example of the mutual benefits you and your baby receive from one another.)

COMFORT

What to Do

- ❏ Use Abdominal Effleurage (page 40).
- ❏ Use The Balloon relaxation technique below.
- ❏ Use Airflow Relaxation (page 164).
- ❏ Do not take aspirin or ibuprofen during postpartum or while nursing.

LABOR TIPS

The Balloon is an excellent technique for relaxing your pelvic area during a long, difficult labor. This can be a real help if you've hit a plateau and are making little or no progress. This kind of problem usually results from a number of factors but, no matter how it starts, it can create a great deal of tension within you, and that tension can prolong the plateau. Balloon relaxation will help you move that tension out of your body so that you can work unimpeded to give birth to your baby.

RELAXATION TECHNIQUES

THE BALLOON

Benefits: Relaxes and relieves pain, especially of the abdominal muscles.

1. Rest in a reclining or a semi-reclining position.
2. Gently place your hands on your lower abdomen, just above the pubic bone.
3. Position your arms so that the fingers of each hand point toward the midline of your body, and your elbows are resting comfortably on the bed, chair, or pillow.

4. Gently close your eyes and take a deep, relaxing sigh.
5. Begin breathing slowly and easily, and imagine that your hands are resting on a balloon.
6. As you inhale, notice how the balloon effortlessly fills with air.
7. Exhale and feel the balloon spontaneously deflate.
8. Continue experiencing the movements of the balloon as it slowly fills with air as you inhale, and gently lets go of the air as you exhale.
9. Notice the changing shape and size of the balloon. What color is it? Watch the color lighten as the balloon fills with air, and darken as the air flows out.
10. As the balloon gently inflates and deflates, notice the muscles of your abdomen rising and falling beneath your fingers.
11. Feel the muscles soften and relax each time the balloon goes limp.
12. Notice how warm your abdomen feels under your fingers.
13. Continue to rest and relax as you observe the soft, limp, warm feeling in your belly with each exhalation.

AIRFLOW RELAXATION

Benefits: Relaxes abdominal and vaginal area to relieve discomfort of involution.

1. Rest in a comfortable position, with your eyes closed. Begin with a deep, relaxing sigh.
2. Breathe slowly and easily, concentrating on your exhalations. Exhale through your mouth or nose—it doesn't matter as long as you focus on exhaling.
3. Feel the total relaxation that comes each time the air flows out of your body, taking all the tension with it.
4. Now, try to redirect the airflow so that it seems to leave your body through the vaginal opening, instead of your mouth or nose. Imagine the air passing from your lungs down through your abdomen and uterus, out through the cervix, and on out through the vagina.
5. Continue relaxing and letting the air flow out through your vagina for as long as needed.

Comments: As you do this exercise, you'll feel your belly soften and relax. Your vagina will feel open and loose, and you may notice a sensation of warmth and tingling or coolness in this area. If you have difficulty imagining air flowing in a particular direction, try to see it in your mind. When I do this exercise, I often imagine the air as soft, blue lines, like the ones cartoonists draw to represent the wind blowing. If you can't "see" it, try to feel it or hear it as it flows through your body.

(*See also* Vaginal Discharge, below.)

Vaginal Discharge

Before you became pregnant, your uterus prepared each month to receive and care for a fertilized egg. This process involved the formation of a thick, soft, blood-rich lining that would serve as a nutritious nest for a growing baby. In the months when you didn't conceive, this lining disintegrated and became the menstrual flow. After you became pregnant, the fertilized egg embedded itself into this thick lining, tapping into your blood supply for nutrients and oxygen. Part of this lining also helped form the placenta, which continued to nourish your baby until birth.

Because this special uterine lining is no longer needed, it will disintegrate during postpartum and be expelled by your body. This cast-off tissue, along with the blood from the site where the placenta peeled off of your uterine wall, compose a vaginal discharge called *lochia.* The flow of lochia will be quite heavy the first few days, after which it will decrease gradually until it disappears in three to four weeks. The amount of lochia will vary throughout the day. It usually increases during or after fundal massage and when you stand up after lying down for a while. You may have less discharge at night when you are lying down, but may notice a gush of lochia just after standing up in the morning.

In the beginning the lochia is bright red, but by the end of the first week it will have faded to a brown, rusty color. The color will gradually lighten, and by about the tenth day it will be a whitish yellow. The discharge will slowly dwindle until it's completely gone. If you aren't nursing your baby, your next period will probably start two to four weeks later. If you are nursing, you may not have any periods until your baby is weaned.

COMFORT

What to Do

❑ Use a sanitary napkin to absorb the lochia.

❑ If your doctor has advised against tub baths until the lochia stops, you can use a sitz bath to cleanse your vaginal area and give you a feeling of freshness. (A sitz bath means you sit your bottom in a small tub of very warm water. The hospital may have given you a plastic sitz tub to take home. If not, you can buy one at a pharmacy.)

❑ Notify your birth attendant if the lochia has a foul odor, or if the discharge causes you to burn or itch. (The lochia should have the same odor as your normal menstrual flow.)

What to Avoid

❑ *Do not use tampons.* Your cervix is still partially open and the placental site has not healed, making you vulnerable to infection. A tampon will only add to your vulnerability.

❑ *Do not douche unless your birth attendant recommends it.*

❑ Avoid using vaginal deodorant sprays. They can irritate the delicate tissues of your vagina mucosa, and may make your stitches sting.

Vaginal Soreness

See Vaginal Weakness.

Vaginal Weakness

"The first few days, it felt like everything was loose and sagging down below . . . like there was no support down there."

"I felt open. I don't know any other way to describe it. It felt as though my vagina was wide open and my uterus might fall out at any minute."

During the first days of postpartum, your entire vaginal area may feel loose, or "open," or sore and stretched out of shape. The muscles of your pelvic floor have just undergone several hours of being stretched just about as far as they can go. It's no wonder that all the stress and pressure of childbirth leaves them feeling weak and, sometimes, sore.

You and your husband may worry that your vagina will never regain its former tone and shape, and you may fear the effect this could have on your sexual activity and enjoyment with each other. But, with the right exercise, you can restore good muscle tone to this area.

COMFORT

What to Do

❑ Practice the Kegel exercise (page 28) frequently throughout the day to restore strength and tone to your pelvic floor muscles.
❑ Rest in the Knee-Chest position (page 7) to relieve discomfort.
❑ For soreness, soak in very warm water or apply an ice pack.

What to Avoid

❑ Avoid applying heat if the area is swollen. Consult your birth attendant about swelling or persistent pain.

(*See also* Pelvic Pressure, page 96; Sexual Adjustments, postpartal, page 151; and Stitches, page 155.)

Weight

When you were pregnant, you probably couldn't wait for the day when you'd get rid of all those extra pounds. If so, you might have been dis-appointed that first day after the birth when you weighed yourself. If you're like most new moms, you lost about twelve pounds—the average combined weight of the baby, placenta, amniotic sac, and fluid.

After all those months of gaining weight, it can be a real letdown to realize that much of it is still with you. Looking in the mirror, you finally can see what you look like without the bulk of your baby in front of you. But what you see may confirm your worst fears—your hips are broader and your thighs and waist are thicker than before the pregnancy. Your breasts may also be larger. As you look in the mirror, keep in mind that much of what you see is fluid, which you'll lose in urine and perspiration over the next weeks. Remember, too, that all these changes in your body shape occurred gradually, over a period of nine months. It's only reasonable to expect your body to take a while to return to its previous shape.

By the time you go for your six-weeks check-up, you probably will have lost twenty to twenty-five pounds. If you feel you need to lose more, ask your birth attendant about a sensible weight-loss diet and exercise program.

COMFORT

What to Do

❑ Begin a regular program of exercise and recreation to speed weight loss. Here are some suggestions:

- Take a brisk, half-hour walk daily, gradually increasing the length of time.
- Join a postpartum exercise class. If you had an uncomplicated birth and recuperation, you can begin a standard postpartum exercise class about two or three weeks after the baby is born. Consult your birth attendant before joining a more strenuous program.
- To strengthen and tone specific parts of the body, check for that subject in the prenatal and postpartum sections of the Comfort Guide. For example, you'll find abdominal exercises listed under "Abdominal Weakness" (page 8) in the prenatal section, and leg exercises listed under "Leg Cramps" (page 43).

❑ See "Weight Gain," (page 115) for information and tips on nutritious eating.

What to Avoid

❑ Do not start a weight-loss diet until after you've weaned your baby from the breast.

(*See also* Abdominal Weakness, page 8).

Index